HOW DOES LAETRILE WORK?

Laetrile advocates are deeply divided about what exactly Laetrile does—whether it cures cancer, prevents it, or simply controls it—or how, precisely, it works its alleged wonders. But that there are wonders, they agree on most passionately. Dr. Richardson claims that patient after patient reports essentially the same story: Laetrile has lessened their pain, increased their appetite, improved their appearance, made them, in short, feel better—something other therapies have failed to do.

The medical establishment responds by saying that Laetrile patients are merely experiencing the classic effects of any placebo. A sugar pill, they say, would have done the same . . .

The clash between the American medical establishment and practitioners of unorthodox cancer therapy goes on, unresolved . . .

CASE # 122

Mrs. Thelma Mosca (case 122) was diagnosed as having cancer of the cervix in January of 1975 and was slated for surgery including a radical hysterectomy. She changed her mind about the surgery and decided to try Laetrile instead. At this point her doctor told her she would be dead within three months. Two years after beginning Laetrile therapy, she is leading an active and rewarding life of involvement in community service.

CASE # 150

Shane Horton (case 150) was six years old when he developed osteosarcoma of the right upper arm and of the spine. This was confirmed both by X-ray and bone-marrow biopsy. His doctors advised that there was no hope. It was at this point that his parents elected Laetrile therapy. Three years after beginning Laetrile therapy, all evidence of bone cancer had vanished, and Shane was enjoying the life of a completely normal nine-year-old.

CASE # 107

John Peterson (case 107) had been given less than a year to live as a result of inoperable cancer of the prostate. His disease progressed rapidly, causing intense and constant pain. His body jerked in spasms, he began bleeding from the rectum, and often passed out from pain and weakness. It was at this point that he turned to Laetrile. Within 30 days of his first injection he was able to drive his own car and lead a near-normal life.

CASE # 152

Mrs. Lorette Lau (case 152) was told by her doctor in 1975 that, unless she submitted to radiation or chemotherapy as treatment for her cancer of the ovary, she could not live longer than a year. She declined his advice and came to the Richardson Clinic for metabolic therapy instead. She has responded beautifully and continues to enjoy good health.

CASE # 115

Mrs. Lorraine Ford (case 115) suffered from inoperable cancer of the liver, with previous cancer of the breast. Statistically, most patients in this category are dead within six months of diagnosis. After the failure of chemotherapy, she turned to Laetrile as a last resort in December of 1974. Today she leads an active and normal life.

Laetrile Case Histories

The Richardson Cancer Clinic Experience

John A. Richardson, M.D.
& Patricia Griffin, R.N.

With a Special Introduction
to the Bantam Edition
by Robert Sam Anson

BANTAM BOOKS
Toronto / New York / London

This low-priced Bantam Book has been completely reset in a type face designed for easy reading, and was printed from new plates. It contains the complete text of the original hard-cover edition.
NOT ONE WORD HAS BEEN OMITTED.

LAETRILE CASE HISTORIES: THE RICHARDSON CANCER CLINIC EXPERIENCE
A Bantam Book / published by arrangement with American Media

PRINTING HISTORY
American Media edition published May 1977
2nd printing .... June 1977
Bantam edition / June 1977

ISBN 0-553-11491-3

Published simultaneously in the United States and Canada

Bantam Books are published by Bantam Books, Inc. Its trademark, consisting of the words "Bantam Books" and the portrayal of a bantam, is registered in the United States Patent Office and in other countries. Marca Registrada. Bantam Books, Inc., 666 Fifth Avenue, New York, New York 10019.

PRINTED IN THE UNITED STATES OF AMERICA

Dedicated to
Ernst T. Krebs, Jr., Ph.D.
and to the
memory of
his father
Ernst T. Krebs, Sr., M.D.
and his brother
Byron Krebs, M.D.
pioneers in the development
and use of Laetrile

"Only science which has lost faith in itself must use power instead of reason to convince others."

Nicholas Von Hoffman
KNX Radio
March 3, 1977

Contents

Special Introduction to the Bantam Edition

by Robert Sam Anson

They come, most of them, because, quite simply, they have no place left to go. They have done the course: radiation, surgery, chemotherapy, immunotherapy, all that American medicine has to offer, and, at best, it has only delayed their date with death. And now, as death approaches, either with no hope left, or fearful of yet more rounds with the surgeon's knife, they have come to a clinic in Tijuana, and a treatment which their government and the American medical establishment has labeled as worthless, a fraud and a hoax. It doesn't matter to them now. They are willing to try anything, even so remote a possibility as being injected with a substance made from nothing more exotic than apricot seeds: They have nothing to lose. The thing that is killing them is cancer.

The desperate trek to the Laetrile clinics in Mexico, Germany, and the United States have been going on now more than twenty years. Last year alone, more than 20,000 Americans made the trip. Statistically, the odds are overwhelming that the journey for most of them will be in vain. Their cancers will still kill them. But maybe less quickly. Maybe less painfully. Maybe, some of them think, not at all. That is why they come, ignoring the advice of their doctors, chancing harassment from their government. To take the pills, and receive the injections of the amber-colored substance called Laetrile. And, in the process, perhaps get some hope.

Hope, however slim or unwarranted, is the one sure property of "amygdalin," the proper name for the chemical extracted from the apricot and peach kernels, bitter almonds and many other plants and seeds. That hope—the utter conviction in many Laetrile advocates—that amygdalin retards, cures or even prevents cancer is what has kept people going to Mexico, and the controversy over Laetrile alive for more than twenty-five years.

Because Laetrile is a medical outlaw. Until its recent legalization by a handful of states, to sell or import it anywhere in the United States was a criminal offense. Federal agencies still ban Laetrile. Those who sell or import it into the United States, whatever their motive or medical credentials, can be charged with a felony, punishable by up to a year in prison, and/or a $10,000 fine. The prosecutions have not stopped the determined from getting Laetrile, or diminished the substance's appeal. What it has done is create a thriving black market, and driven up the price of illegally imported Laetrile several times over its cost in Mexico. Laetrile's very illicitness has, if anything, enhanced its reputation among cancer patients—and made martyrs of the Laetrile activists who risk importing it.

The primary issue—whether Laetrile actually works—has widened to embrace far more fundamental questions. Does the government have the right to protect its people from a cure which it believes worthless—especially when proven cancer-*causers,* such as cigarettes, are perfectly legal? Should citizens, particularly the terminally ill, have freedom of choice in selecting the therapy which they believe will help them best? Are there vested interests which control American medicine? Has, in fact, American medicine been doing all it can to find a cure for cancer?

Emotions about Laetrile are running so high that at a recent FDA-sponsored conference about the substance in Kansas City, a doctor who asked the audience, "Do you really think that a quarter million physicians would let people die because they want to make money off them?" was greeted with angry choruses of "Yes, yes, yes."

It is an unlikely battle, waged over an unlikely substance. On one side is arrayed the whole of the American medical establishment: the Food and Drug Administration, the National Cancer Institute, the American Cancer Society, the American Medical Association, and such prestigious cancer research centers as New York's Sloan-Kettering Institute, all of whom claim to have found—to use the words of an FDA position paper—"no acceptable scientific evidence that Laetrile has any anti-cancer effect."

On the other rampart are the equally determined Laetrile forces: Laetrile patients themselves (an estimated 200,000 Americans have been treated with the substance), their organized lobbies (chief among them, VOCAL-*VICTORY OVER CANCER ACTION LEAGUE,* the International Association of Cancer Victims and Friends, the Cancer Control Society, and the Committee for Freedom of Choice in Cancer Therapy), and a scattered number of private doctors, biochemists and researchers, a number of whom have used Laetrile and been prosecuted, fined, even jailed for their troubles.

The chasm between the two groups is enormous, the rhetoric of both sides highly charged. "Goddamn quackery," the chief spokesman for the California branch of the American Cancer Society calls Laetrile. "Premeditated murderers in the first degree," a Laetrile activist terms the authorities who ban it.

There is not even agreement on what Laetrile is, much less what it does. According to the FDA, Laetrile is a "new drug," and thus falls under the provisions of the Food, Drug and Cosmetic Act of 1962, which bans the importation and sale of drugs which have not been proven safe and effective. Not a drug at all, counter the Laetrile advocates; amygdalin is a vitamin, "Vitamin B_{17}," a substance which the FDA and the rest of the medical establishment insists does not exist.

For Laetrile to be made available, the authorities

argue, it must first be certified as valuable through testing on laboratory animals—just as twenty-seven other anti-cancer drugs have been certified. "Laetrile," an FDA position paper states, "is the most-tested cancer drug in history." And every test has resulted in failure. Since the first study conducted by the California Medical Association in 1953, through those sponsored by the National Cancer Institute between 1957 and 1975, to the most recent series at Sloan-Kettering and other cancer research centers; more than a dozen different experiments in all, have all come up with the same result: Laetrile is worthless; indeed, worse than worthless, since those who turn to it, often turn away from traditional therapy which might extend, even save their lives. As Dr. Daniel Martin, who has tested Laetrile, puts it: "The only thing it can do is take your money." The Laetrile forces rejoin that the testing on amygdalin has been rigged, biased, and, in some instances, outright fraudulent. They present animal test data of their own—notably an initial study conducted at Sloan-Kettering in 1972–73 on cancerous mice by senior researcher Dr. Kanematsu Sugiura, who concluded that "amygdalin significantly inhibits the appearance of lung metastases"—along with numerous case histories and personal testimonials, which the medical establishment dismisses as "anecdotal" and thus not scientifically valid.

Each side questions the motives of the other. The medical establishment charges that the Laetrile activists are charlatans and fast-buck artists. A spokesman for the National Cancer Institute says their trade is "a wicked business, on a par with swindling widows." In turn, many Laetrile proponents see the government, the health bureaucracy and the drug companies joined in a vast, genocidal, even international conspiracy against cancer victims. Not long ago, *American Opinion,* the official publication of the John Birch Society, a number of whose members are joined in the Laetrile cause, reported: "Laetrile therapists fear that the conspiratorial plan may now be for the U.S. government (possibly by way of Sloan-Kettering), the United Nations and Communist Russia suddenly to discover a 'new' control for cancer, which would be Laetrile under another name—so that the conspirators would get the credit. It would increase the difficulty of fighting the Communists if they are credited with defeating cancer." To be sure, some of the charges coming from the government have been equally unsupported. In at least one criminal case against a Laetrile doctor, the government subsequently admitted that one of its witnesses had knowingly perjured himself. "We are going to fight dirty now," a spokesman for the American Cancer Society recently told a reporter.

The passion that surrounds Laetrile—indeed, any purported treatment for cancer—is understandable. The disease does not lend itself to rationality. For all the reassuring messages from the American Cancer Society (an "emergency" organization created to combat cancer in 1913) about "curing cancer in your lifetime" and cancer being "one of the most curable of diseases," cancer remains frustratingly, maddeningly mysterious. Moreover, despite the billions of dollars that have been poured into traditional cancer research in the last twenty years (nearly $900 million committed by the government this year alone), and continued predictions that the cure for cancer is just around the symbolic corner, the reality is that scant more is known about the cause, working and ultimate riddance of cancer than was when Hippocrates, the father of modern medicine, identified *karkinos* (the Greek word for crab) twenty-four centuries ago.

All that is certain is that cancer remains a rapacious killer. One of every four people alive now—one of four people reading these words—will eventually get cancer in one form or another (there are more than 150 varieties), and one in six will die from it. Last year, more than 600,000 Americans contracted cancer, and more than half that number died from it, making cancer the second leading killer in the United States, just behind diseases of the heart. And the disease grows more deadly year after year. In 1930, the cancer death rate among Americans was 112 per 100,000; by 1950, it had climbed to 125 per 100,000; fourteen years later, it had risen to 132 per 100,000.

The most depressing statistics, however, are those for survival five years after treatment. Ironically, the sharpest advance in longevity rates occurred before the 1950s, at a time when funds for cancer research were modest, and treatment relatively unsophisticated. Even then, a number of experts ascribe the progress to transfusions and antibiotics, which enabled cancer victims to survive not the disease, but the treatments used to cure it. Since the early 50s, according to Nobel-laureate James Watson, whose work in DNA research has extended into cancer, "the cure rates have improved only about 1 per cent." The statistics of the National Cancer Institute, the semi-autonomous, government-supported organization which supervises and conducts nearly all the cancer research in the United States, tend to bear Watson out. Since the 1950s, the cancer survival rate for various forms of cancer, which, taken together, account for 66 per cent of the incidence of the disease, have, according to NCI figures, increased by five percentage points or fewer. The survival rate for lung cancer, one of the biggest killers, has increased only 1 per cent; breast cancer, 4 per cent, while cancer of the colon inched forward also only by 1 per cent. In fact, with some cancers—about 13 per cent of the total—the survival rate has actually *declined* since the 50s. One of those cancers is *cervix uteri,* which is readily detectable by the simple Pap smear test. Yet, despite all the publicity on behalf of Pap smears, and the burgeoning number of women who now have them as a matter of routine, the survival rate for *cervix uteri fell* three percentage points between 1965 and 1969.

The frustration born of such grim figures intensified as Congress, spurred on by the passage of the National Cancer Act of 1971—the legislation that declared "war" on cancer—committed hundreds of millions of dollars a year to research, with little visible effect. "It's not like going to the moon, where, if you have a crash program, and spend a lot of money, you know that you are going to get there," says one prominent cancer researcher. "The fact is, we don't know much about cancer, and money alone won't tell us. It's like going to the moon without knowing Newton's laws of gravity." Watson is even more blunt. The national cancer program, he says flatly, "is bunk."

Bunk or not, billions continue to be spent, and nearly all of them on refining traditional, well-established treatments—notably surgery, radiation and chemotherapy—none of which have yet achieved a breakthrough. By the nature of the profession, the medical establishment is instinctively conservative, cautious, and, in the opinion of a number of critics, demonstrably hostile to untried or unorthodox solutions. The Pap smear test, for instance, was available fifteen years before the American Medical Association gave it its blessing, and it became common practice. The professional jealousies among researchers are notorious, and there is intense competition for limited funds. As a result, most cancer research hews to the tried and true. A scientist at the National Cancer Institute explained the dilemma in a recent interview: "Look, when you've got ten thousand radiologists and millions of dollars' worth of radiation equipment, you give radiation treatments, even if study after study shows that a lot of it does more harm than good. What else are they going to do? They're doing what they have been trained to do. Like the surgeons. They've been trained to cut, so they cut."

As the cutting and radiating and drugging continues, it becomes more expensive. Bills of $40,000 and upward for sophisticated cancer treatment at centers like Sloan-Kettering are not uncommon. Even then, there is no guarantee of success. Oftentimes, in fact, treatments for advanced cancer can seem worse than the disease. Massive surgery, such as radical mastectomies for breast cancer, or castration for testicular cancer, leaves the patients mutilated and despondent. Radiation can cause burns and scarring, and lead to total loss of body hair, not to mention an increased incidence of other forms of cancer. So, too, chemotherapy has dangerous side effects, while immunotherapy, the latest and, in the opinion of many experts, most promising of the traditional approaches, can expose the body to the ravages of other disease.

Taken together, the frustration, the emotion, the pain and expense—the plain terror that cancer uniquely engenders—have found their climactic release in the substance known as Laetrile. Here is a substance, its proponents claim, which is cheaper, safer and far more effective than anything "orthodox medicine," as they call it, has yet come up with, for all the billions they have spent. The Laetrile advocates themselves are deeply divided about what exactly Laetrile does—whether it cures cancer, prevents it, or simply controls it—or how, precisely, it works its alleged wonders. But that there are wonders, all pro-Laetrile people agree most passionately. Patient after patient who has made the trek to Laetrile clinics come back with essentially the same story: Laetrile has lessened their pain, increased their appetite, improved their appearance, made them, in short, feel better—something other therapies have failed to do.

The medical establishment responds that Laetrile patients are merely experiencing the classic effects of any placebo. A sugar pill, they say, would have done the same. To prove their case, they point to a study conducted by the Mayo Clinic, which found that 112 of 288 cancer patients—about 39 per cent—reported a diminishing of at least half their pain, after being treated with nothing more than sugar pills.

Laetrile is not the first substance over which the American medical establishment and practitioners of unorthodox cancer therapy have clashed. In the 50s, the battle was over the Gerson diet, devised by a New York doctor named Max Gerson. Gerson claimed that most cancers had nutritional roots. The AMA declared him a quack, and lifted his license to practice. Albert Schweitzer, whose wife Gerson treated, later called Gerson "a medical genius who walked among us." In the 60s, the fight was over Krebiozen, a supposed cancer-curing drug championed by Dr. Andrew Ivy, until then one of the most respected men in medicine. Ivy was subsequently arrested on 240 counts of violating the drug laws. After a trial that lasted 289 days, the jury found him innocent of every charge, said that they believed that Krebiozen had merit, and urged the FDA to test it. The FDA refused, and Ivy was ruined. Krebiozen, meanwhile, quietly disappeared.

There have been other encounters, some of them serious, most merely frivolous; but none can compare with the confrontation over Laetrile. For one thing, Laetrile has been on the scene longer, and been taken by more people, than any of the other unorthodox treatments. Amygdalin was first isolated from bitter almonds by a pair of French chemists in 1830. More than a hundred years later, in 1935, a San Francisco physician named Ernst Krebs, Sr., began the first experiments with amygdalin as a cancer cure. The trouble with Kreb's first formulation, aside from its debatable efficacy, was its toxicity; the ground apricot seeds, in extraordinary concentration, were rich in cyanide, one of the deadliest substances known to man. It was left to Krebs' son, Ernst, Jr., a biochemist, to purify amygdalin, remove its toxicity, and rechristen it Laetrile.

Krebs Jr.'s discovery came in 1952. A year later, the first public testing on it was done under the auspices of the California Medical Association, the results of which led the State Department of Health to forbid its use in California. Thus, Laetrile moved south, below the border to Tijuana. There, in two private clinics, where patients averaged a three-week, $1,500 stay (including room and board), Laetrile was administered to a small, if devoted following.

But for the intense interest of Andrew McNaughton, a charismatic, highly controversial Canadian, Laetrile therapy might have languished. But McNaughton had a marked propensity for attaching himself to unorthodox, unpopular causes, from gun-running (initially for the Israelis, later for Castro) to high-risk financial ventures, one of which resulted in his conviction for conspiracy to manipulate Pan American mine stocks. He was sentenced to one year in jail and fined $25,000. On appeal, the sentence was reduced to one day in jail and a $10,000 fine.

The son of a Canadian war hero, and himself a highly decorated test pilot, McNaughton was drawn into Laetrile through a chance meeting with Krebs Jr. in a Florida drugstore in 1956. The two men talked, and McNaughton became intrigued with Krebs's theories, so much so that he soon threw his energies, along with most of his fortune, into the Laetrile cause. He created the McNaughton Foundation in Canada for the promotion of Laetrile, and, when success eluded him, moved to California. Stymied again, he shifted his operations to Tijuana. Meanwhile, interest in Laetrile—which soon spread to twenty-six other foreign countries besides Mexico—increased, as did the federal authorities' interest in McNaughton. He was arrested the first time for smuggling Laetrile into the United States in 1971, less than a year after the FDA had denied his application to do research on the substance. The charges against him were dropped, at the request of the government, for lack of evidence. McNaughton was arrested again in 1976, this time in the company of a number of other Laetrile activists, including Dr. John A. Richardson, and charged with conspiring to smuggle Laetrile into the United States, a far more serious offense. At the time of this writing, McNaughton has not yet been brought to trial, and it becomes increasingly likely that he never will.

Over the years, other doctors and private individuals had been arrested for similar offenses. Their cases, however, went almost without notice. McNaughton and Richardson, because of their prominence in the Laetrile movement, were an entirely different story. Their arrests loosed massive publicity about Laetrile, and heightened public awareness about the unorthodox therapy. Much of the publicity focused on McNaughton's highly visible past (one of the contributors to his foundation was New Jersey Mafia boss "Bayonne Joe" Zicarelli, who donated $130,000 after his sister had been treated with Laetrile), his alleged wealth (which McNaughton denied, claiming he could not even afford a lawyer) and the conservative associations of Dr. Richardson and other prominent Laetrile activists, a number of whom were members of the John Birch Society. With his father, Krebs Jr. had also been convicted of interstate shipment of another drug, "Vitamin B_{15}," which allegedly improved the performance of athletes and race horses.

Negative as much of the publicity was, it aroused the interest of thousands of cancer patients, who seemed to care less about a man's political beliefs than about a potential cure he was offering for their suffering.

But politics could not be removed from Laetrile entirely, especially after Richardson's arrest. For Richardson is politically active in conservative causes, and those causes quickly rallied to his support. The Birch Society itself took no official position on Laetrile, but Birch Society members, along with other conservative activists came forward to play important leadership roles in the organizations that sprang up to lobby and proselytize on behalf of Laetrile. They published newsletters and showed films to civic groups. There were T-shirts and bumper stickers, proclaiming "Apricot Power," and, most importantly, intensive lobbying in corridors and offices in virtually every statehouse in the country.

Their strategy was basic: if the FDA could not be moved, they would outflank it. Let the federal government continue to ban Laetrile, they reasoned; the states would be easier to move. Once the pressure at the grassroots level became intolerable, the federal government would have to yield.

And, to a remarkable extent, the Laetrile activisits succeeded. By June 1977, eight states had approved the use of Laetrile in one form or another, invariably by lopsided margins, and fifteen other states have similar measures pending.

The experiences in Indiana are typical. There, Laetrile was opposed by both the Democratic and Republican legislative leaderships, the politically potent Indiana Medical Association, the faculty of the Indiana University Medical School (the largest in the country), and Republican Governor Otis Bowen, a physician, who announced at the outset that he would veto any law legalizing Laetrile. They never had a chance. The House adopted the bill 85 to 10; the Senate followed suit by a margin of 44 to 4. And when Bowen, fulfilling his pledge, vetoed the bill, his veto was easily overridden.

What the Laetrile advocates had done was organize. The statehouse halls were filled with placard-carrying, chanting demonstrators. A petition was presented with 44,000 signatures. As the Governor himself ruefully put it: "Every time a senator or representative stuck his head out the door, they were after him. I got clobbered." Even the executive director of the Indiana Medical Association was impressed. "I wish they would be on my side," he said, "if I ever want something passed."

The argument that the Laetrile forces presented in Indiana, and continue to present elsewhere, boils down to a deceptively simple notion: namely, people who are dying have the right to do so on their own terms, and select any therapy *they* think will work.

So far, at least, the argument has proved difficult to resist. This past May, a federal district judge in Oklahoma, Luther Bohannon, ruled that a terminally ill cancer patient named Glen L. Rutherford—along with all other cancer patients who produced affadavits from their doctors stating that their cases were terminal—could import Laetrile for his own use. Bohannon further ruled that the FDA had been arbitrary in banning the substance, and, indeed, had not even properly demonstrated that it had jurisdiction over Laetrile. A month earlier, another terminally ill cancer patient, Joseph Rizzo of Brooklyn, had obtained a similar order from another federal district court, allowing him to use Laetrile during a thirty-day test period. At the end of the test period, Rizzo's physician, Dr. Baldassare B. Cumella, was guardedly optimistic. "Laetrile will not cure cancer," Cumella said, "but it will enable a cancer victim to die in dignity and not in misery." According to Cumella, his patient had been freed of much of his previous pain, and had regained sufficient strength to leave his bed and even take short walks every day. Cumella also speculated that Rizzo's longevity may have also been extended by several months. "The improvement so far," he concluded, "has been impressive."

The increasing public pressure for Laetrile, however carefully orchestrated, has produced cracks in the cancer establishment's once solid wall of opposition to Laetrile. The most notable defection in recent years has been Dr. Dean Burk, the former head of the National Cancer Institute's cytochemistry section, and now a prominent pro-Laetrile spokesman. While at NCI, Burk attacked a study on Laetrile sponsored by the Institute, charging that its testing procedures were sloppy and biased, its data twisted, and that rather than disproving Laetrile's effectiveness, they actually substantiated the case. The cancer establishment's opposition to the substance, Burk said, "lacks, in my judgment, sound scientific, medical and constitutionally legal basis, and is perhaps suggestive of the attitude of Aesop's dog in the manger."

At Sloan-Kettering, whose experiments have been cited both by anti- and pro-Laetrile forces to buttress their arguments, a rump newsletter, entitled *Second Opinion,* has sprung up, denouncing the center for an alleged "Laetrile cover-up." Asserting that it represents the voice of "rank and file employees" of the center, *Second Opinion* charges that "the top leaders of SKI are terrified of reporting *any* positive results with Laetrile even if these are modified by more negative findings."

In fact, Sloan-Kettering has recently released a complete report based on four years of testing Laetrile in animals. According to spokesmen for the Institute, they found no evidence that Laetrile cures or prevents cancer, or is beneficial in treating malignant tumors.

No doubt the Laetrile advocates will not be satisfied. All the Sloan-Kettering tests, indeed, nearly all the orthodox Laetrile experiments, have been conducted on animals, namely mice, and many Laetrile proponents insist that the substance's true effect shows up only on human beings. Whether testing is done on animals or humans, there are a number of important variables. Tests yield statistics, and statistics can be read and interpreted—or, for that matter, juggled—according to personal preference. The Laetrile forces contend that the cancer establishment has been doing just that. Other scientifically accepted tests, notably the 1953 study in California, are suspect because of the credentials of the researchers. In the California experiments, for instance, the doctors who found no value in Laetrile were later accused of being paid $50,000 each by the American Tobacco Institute. Indeed, one of the doctors proclaimed "a pack a day keeps cancer away." As it happens, he later died of lung cancer, while his colleague died in a fire where smoking in bed was suspected as the cause.

Even researchers of the highest probity can run into trouble. Sloan-Kettering's Sugiura, who caused such a stir by finding that Laetrile inhibited the spread of cancerous tumors in mice, was later unable to repeat his experiments. The reason, Sloan-Kettering officials suspect, is that in the first experiment, Sugiura knew which animals were being injected with Laetrile; the second time, he did not. According to some pro-Laetrile advocates, the reason is that the batch of Laetrile used for the second test was of questionable origin, purity, and age. The Laetrile forces have also had their problems. Dr. Ernesto Contreras, the director of Centro Medico del Mar, the largest Laetrile clinic in Tiajuana, submitted, at the request of the FDA, the case histories of twelve of his patients. The dosages he administered at this early stage of using Laetrile were much smaller than dosages given today, and it appears that there was no follow-up on patients after they left Dr. Contreras's clinic to determine whether or not they continued taking Laetrile. Of the nine patients who could be located, six had died of cancer, another had succumbed to a different disease, and the cancer of yet another had spread. The ninth man reported he was feeling fine. The difficulty is, he had been treated with other cancer therapies, in addition to Laetrile. Thus, it was impossible to conclude which treatment had made him better.

In short, not all testing is as scientifically pristine as it appears to be. Yet, until recently, the medical establishment has been unwilling to test Laetrile further, or to observe its effects on human beings. Now, because of growing public pressure, that attitude is changing dramatically. The National Cancer Institute, which previously insisted that "not one shred of evidence" existed that Laetrile had any effect on cancer, has announced that it is "seriously considering" testing Laetrile on volunteer cancer patients. Dr. Lewis Thomas, president of Sloan-Kettering, agrees that such tests, while unprecedented in cancer research, have to be undertaken, and that the matter is most urgent. There have been similar calls for such testing from other respected sources and medical journals, all of whom, however, preface their recommendations with expressions of confidence that Laetrile will be found to be worthless.

Is it? That, of course, is the outstanding question, and the reason that this book has been written. That it is being written at all is perhaps the best proof that Dr. Thomas is correct when he terms the controversy evoked by Laetrile "unprecedented." There has rarely, if ever, been a medical debate so heated, with the basic facts so disputed, the motives of the participants on both sides so called into question. Of course, there has never been a disease quite like cancer.

We are used to science that provides us with precise, definitive answers. Something is either true or not true. A cure works or it doesn't work. Unfortunately, there are, as yet, not those sorts of answers available about Laetrile. For perhaps the first time, the layman is left to fend almost entirely for himself. If he relies on the word of the organized, established medical community which insists that their tests have been thorough, fair and exhaustive—he can only conclude that Laetrile is without value. If, on the other hand, he is moved by the arguments of Dr. Richardson and his allies, the case histories and testimonials of Laetrile patients themselves, and still other tests, such as experiments conducted inIsrael, Indonesia, and West Germany—then he will conclude that Laetrile is worth trying.

The choice comes down to where one places one's trust and belief—perhaps how desperately one *needs* to believe, when the disease is cancer.

The arguments put forth by both sides are compelling. Freedom of choice versus medical chaos; scientific data versus human experience; the traditional versus the unorthodox. And, on the narrow middle ground, agreement on one fundamental truth: Cancer is still killing us, and we don't know why.

The book you are about to read puts forth one of those arguments, and does so powerfully. But, however convincing, it is only one argument, one segment of a still elusive truth. Many people will dispute Dr. Richardson's thesis, and his conclusions. That they ought to be read, pondered and critically evaluated cannot be denied.

For, if one fact has emerged from our battle with cancer, it is how little we know about it. With this book, we know more.

Foreword

In no other aspect of medicine are families so deeply divided as they are in the matter of treatment of cancer. Uncle Joe, who hasn't had any interest in Aunt Harriet in the last thirty years, suddenly becomes deeply involved, rants and raves, and even threatens the doctor with a lawsuit if Harriet chooses unorthodox cancer therapy.

Within the profession itself, peer review groups pass judgment against any physician who deviates from the norm of *accepted* practice, no matter how successful he may be in restoring the health of his patients. *Conformity, not results, is the goal.*

Putting it mildly, it is an interesting world to live in if you are a doctor who happens to believe, as I do, that scientific truth is determined neither by majority vote nor governmental edict.

Until now, the most devastating statement our critics could make about Laetrile is that it is a great theory except for the fact that there is no evidence to support it. Then they usually cite a long list of alleged scientific experiments which have failed to confirm the effectiveness of Laetrile. As my good friend Ed Griffin has pointed out in his excellent book *World Without Cancer; The Story of Vitamin B_{17}*, however, every one of these experiments either utilized inadequate doses, improper criteria, or actually *did* show favorable results after all. Still, the defenders of the *status quo* continue to repeat their convincingly pious chant that there is no evidence.

May the publication of this book at least spare us the repetition of that monotonous claim.

JOHN A. RICHARDSON, M.D.

February 18, 1977

Acknowledgments

As a practicing physician with an extremely heavy patient load (to say nothing of a busy court calendar), I have had little time or patience for writing. Consequently, this book never could have been completed without the help and cooperation of many friends. Clearly the driving force throughout has been Pat Griffin, who has spent literally hundreds of hours poring over records, contacting patients, verifying data, and writing the case summaries themselves. Ed Griffin's section on orthodox medicine has given to this study that full dimension of scholarship that we all have come to expect from his pen and has added greatly to an understanding of the larger picture. My wife, Julie, has been a deep well, supplying unlimited waters of support, understanding, and courage, even in the face of the most bitter odds.

To Ralph Bowman, who not only introduced the subject of Laetrile, but who has been the trusty Sancho in this Don Quixote joust with ancient wrongs, and who, with a constant, seemingly inexhaustible, energy managed the office, masterminded the details, and coped with the unending problems; and, of course, to his wonderful wife, Dolly, who has tolerated us both.

To Mary Botelho, the lone survivor of my original staff, faithful to the end, who, with a congenital eyesight defect, has read more than anyone else in the office.

To Angela Gillmer, R.N., who left the security of orthodoxy to join our cause. To Janice Eby, my trusted and efficient secretary; to Joie Toyotome our expert insurance girl; to my son Stephen, who helped absorb some of the vindictive blows from the arrogant bureaucracy; and to my daughter Becky, our efficiency expert. To Gail and Laura Bowman, Jannell Garrett, Ingrid Davis, Trudy Prince and Joanna Ketner, all faithful toilers in the field. To Matt Bowman, who always carries our orders "right now". To Bela Veress, who keeps up the building; to John "L" Marthaler, whose doctrinally oriented Constitutional approach to the law repeatedly has saved us from the capricious whims of public servants. To Michelle Mahoney, who met the challenge of locating many "long lost" patients; and to John and Astrid Chase, who helped us when we needed it most. To Charlotte Anderson and Margie Gross, my nurses at the time of the first "hit".

To the members of Project Nine; and to Robert Welch who provided the first sensible approach to a theory of cancer in the individual and in a civilization.

To my patients whose personal battles constitute the real drama of this book, I give my heartfelt and eternal thanks.

To the wonderful Grace of God which supplied the logistics for this expedition, not because we deserved it but because of Grace itself.

JOHN A. RICHARDSON, M.D.

March 15, 1977

INTRODUCTION

by Patricia Griffin, R.N., B.S.

I was totally unprepared for my first visit to the Richardson Clinic. As a nurse, I had spent considerable time on cancer wards and I knew what to expect: the awful odor of decaying flesh and the sallow faces of forlorn patients who have been condemned to a sub-human existence as they await their inevitable fate.

No one likes to be in the presence of death and, because there is so little that orthodox medicine can do other than mask the pain with mind-dulling drugs, the doctor and nurse often avoid the terminal cancer patient as much as is ethically acceptable. Examinations are brief. Conversation is kept to a minimum. Where possible, the patient is assigned to staff subordinates. Cancer wards and cancer clinics all are pretty much the same: impersonal, smelly, and depressing.

It was to my amazement, therefore, to discover that the Richardson Clinic did not fit this morbid pattern. The first thing that struck me was that the patients awaiting treatment were engaged in animated conversation. They were talking, not only about their illness but about their children and grandchildren, about the cross-country sightseeing trip they had planned just as soon as they felt strong enough, and of their ultimate return to work. These people were not preoccupied with death; they were planning for life!

Then I noticed the attitude of the staff. They

actually enjoyed being with the patients and spent considerable time with each. They derived genuine satisfaction from learning of the improvement over the previous visit. Their jokes with the patients were not those strained little condescending attempts to be cheerful in the face of tragedy but rather the genuine outbursts of people who were finding fun in their work.

And, finally, I suddenly became aware that the air was completely free from the fetid smell associated with growing cancer.

A middle-aged man stepped from the clinic area into the waiting room and, with a big grin, announced to the patients that this was the last day of treatment for Mrs. So-and-so (everyone responded to the name), that she was headed back to Illinois in the morning, and that everyone was invited to a party to celebrate her departure.

A *party* in a cancer clinic?!

I recalled my days as a student nurse on the bone and joint ward at the University of Michigan Hospital. This was the same picture I had seen there. Sure, the patients had problems—and some of them pretty serious—but it was understood that everyone would get well, or at least return to a near-normal life of health and happiness. In the meantime, spirits usually were high, plans were made for the future, and everyone looked forward to the day of discharge.

When one is trained in and by orthodox medicine as I was, it is difficult to hold an open mind about anything which is contrary to the professional consensus —perhaps even more so than for the non-medically trained layman who at least doesn't have to unlearn old errors to accept new truths. It was natural, therefore, that my first reaction to Laetrile therapy was one of considerable skepticism.

I first heard of Laetrile in 1971 in a health food store. While the concept of cancer's being essentially a deficiency disease appealed to me, I was confident that, if there were any scientific basis to that theory, the great medical research centers would pick it up, thoroughly test it, and then introduce it to mankind *properly*—that is, not through health food stores but through the medical profession itself.

It is a comfortable feeling to have that kind of confidence in one's own profession. And I can relate thoroughly to the mixed emotions of an R.N. who recently came to the Richardson Clinic after her own physician told her bluntly that there was little hope for her recovery. The lady, a Ph.D. in nursing, by the way, because engaged in conversation with a former high school drop-out who was returning for a check-up. He was a fifty-three-year-old Italian bachelor, who had been told at the hospital eight months earlier that he had less than two months to live. Since starting his therapy at the Richardson Clinic, he had regained his former zest for life and, in fact, had just returned from a very successful day at the race track.

It was the nurse's first appointment at the clinic, and she was having second thoughts about being there. Sensing her fear and reluctance, soon the man was explaining to her all about the trophoblastic thesis of cancer, the role of the pancreatic enzymes—and, thus, the need to avoid animal protein in the diet—and the importance of vitamins and minerals of all kinds. When she complained that she couldn't possibly take "all those pills" every day, the high school drop-out said to the nursing Ph.D.: "What do you mean you can't? You came here for help. You've put up with surgery already. A nice lady like you has hair on her face because some doctor screwed up your hormones. Let me tell you how to take those pills. Just put them in your hand a few at a time, pop them into your mouth, and follow with a drink. Of *course* you can do it. And you soon will be feeling thankful to God you did!"

The hardest pill for many professionals to swallow is not the vitamin pill. It is the thought that they have been wrong and, further, that they and their colleagues have strongly criticized those who have been right. How humiliating! There comes a point, after years of administering drugs for almost every human ailment, and after scoffing at "those silly food faddists" for preaching nutrition as an alternative, when the professional finds himself backed into a corner. He has put down drugless medicine so hard and so often that his reputation now is at stake, and he has a vested interest in his own error.

I know because I went through it. It was not easy to accept drugless medicine as a scientifically valid approach to health care. And it especially wasn't easy to let go of all the pet theories about cancer etiology and to view this seemingly complex disease as merely variable manifestations of a single vitamin and enzyme deficiency. But a person can deny reality only so long. My personal experience with patients on Laetrile therapy since 1972 no longer leaves room for skepticism. What I have seen with my own eyes is convincing beyond any doubt. Laetrile *is* effective in the control of human cancer. This book has been prepared so that others can share some of the evidence that has led me to that conclusion.

I feel highly privileged to be able to play a small role in one of the most important and exciting medical revolutions of history. But revolutions are unpleasant. Honorable men on both sides are sacrificed in the ebb and flow of battle. Those that survive often carry the scars of bitterness to their graves. I fervently hope that this study will hasten the day when that revolution is over and when the word cancer will be relegated to the dusty pages of history.

Patricia Griffin, R.N., B.S.
February 15, 1977

I

"You Are Going to Die!"

by John A. Richardson, M.D.

My early years in medical practice; experiences with orthodox cancer therapies; first exposure to the deficiency theory of cancer; meeting with Dr. Ernst T. Krebs, Jr., developer of Laetrile; first results on cancer patients; development and refinement of "metabolic" therapy; importance of recognizing tumors as symptoms of disease, not disease itself; surprise raid and subsequent arrest on June 2, 1972.

Mrs. Evans was almost hysterical when she burst through the door of our clinic. "Look what they did! Look what they did to my car! Just look!"

Two of the men patients followed her back to her car which was parked in front of the clinic and duly reported the damage. While Mrs. Evans had been receiving her injection of Laetrile, someone had permanently scratched on her windshield in large letters: "You are going to die!"

When I heard of the incident, I was dismayed but not surprised. For over a month, a woman had stationed herself conspicuously across the street and had written down the license number of every car that had come to our clinic. Some patients never returned because of it, perhaps feeling that they were going to get into some kind of trouble with the authorities. When the woman was asked why she was recording the license numbers, her reply was candid. She was doing it, she said, for the government and added for emphasis that she was looking forward to the day when all "quack clinics like this will be closed down."

A month or so later, when the license-taking was replaced by photograph-taking, it became clear to us that the state was attempting to frighten away our patients; what it had failed to accomplish through the courts it was now trying to bring about indirectly through intimidation.

But that is jumping into the middle of the story. To understand why and how I came to be the FDA's "public health enemy number one," let us go back to 1971, when it all began.

For over twenty years I had enjoyed a comfortable and satisfying practice in Berkeley, California. Although my specialty was Ear, Nose, and Throat, I considered myself a family-oriented general practitioner and, as such, treated a wide variety of illnesses, including the initial stages of cancer, although the latter on a very limited basis. Over the course of years, I have prescribed all of the currently accepted modalities of cancer treatment: surgery, radiation, and chemotherapy, usually by referral to specialists in these fields. These therapies seldom prolonged the lives of my patients and, in fact, often seemed to shorten them. They hardly seemed worth the cost to the patient either in terms of financial outlay or in suffering from the painful side-effects of radiation burns and drug toxicity. Yet, I took some comfort in the knowledge that what I was prescribing was a "treatment of choice" within the medical profession and that none of my colleagues were obtaining any better results. So I simply did the best I could with what was available—or so I thought.

Then one evening in a local restaurant after dinner with Ralph Bowman—the man who is now my clinic manager and medical assistant—the conversation turned to a substance called Laetrile. Ralph had come across some literature on the subject and began to describe its theoretical action against cancer. I was fascinated immediately at the logic of finding a control for cancer *in nature* and decided to investigate further.

Fortunately, the developers of Laetrile lived right across the bay in San Francisco. Ernst T. Krebs, Sr.,

M.D., had been working with this substance since 1923. His sons, Ernst T. Krebs, Jr., Ph.D., and Byron Krebs, M.D., later joined in the father's research and perfected Laetrile in 1952. I looked up their names in the central telephone directory, and dialed the number. I was pleasantly surprised when an amicable Ernst T. Krebs, Jr., answered the phone and was more than willing to discuss the matter with me at great length.

During the weeks that followed, I read just about everything I could find on the subject and spent many hours at the office of Dr. Krebs discussing the theoretical model as well as the practical application of this substance called Laetrile. It was as though I had returned to medical school, for I found myself boning-up on long-forgotten facts in the field of embryology and biochemistry. The more I learned, the more convinced I became that Dr. Krebs really had the answer.

Basically the theory Krebs advanced is that cancer is not caused by some strange invading force from outside the body, but rather by malfunctions of normal mechanisms solely within the body itself. Those malfunctions are the result of a deficiency in a chemical substance found in certain foods and of a deficiency in certain enzymes produced in the pancreas. The natural chemical food factor is known as nitriloside, or vitamin B_{17}, and the pancreatic enzymes are known as the trypsins.

Vitamin B_{17} is a cyanide-containing compound that gives up its cyanide only in the presence of an enzyme group called beta glucosidase or glucuronidase. But the miracle of nature is that this enzyme group is found to any appreciable extent only in cancer tissue. When it is found elsewhere, it always is accompanied by greater quantities of another enzyme called rhodanese, which has the capacity to convert the cyanide immediately into completely harmless substances. In fact, some of those by-products actually are beneficial to man and play a role in the formation and utilization of other vitamins. Cancer tissue does not have this protecting enzyme. Thus, cancer cells are faced with a double threat; the presence of one enzyme causes them to be exposed to cyanide, while the absence of another enzyme (which is found in all other cells) results in the failure to detoxify.

The net result of this fact of nature is that cancer cells, because of their enzyme composition, are unable to withstand the cyanide from vitamin B_{17} and are destroyed. Normal, non-cancer cells are not threatened by the cyanide and, in fact, are capable of converting it into nutritional substances vital to health. But nature's mechanism will not work if one fails to eat the foods that contain this necessary vitamin, which is exactly what has happened to modern man, whose food supply has become further and further removed from the natural state.

The enzyme factor is equally important, and it is probable that it and the food factor were intended to work together. Basically what happens is this. The enzyme trypsinogen is converted to trypsin in the intestine and there, along with chymotrypsin, is utilized in the digestion of animal protein. The surplus is absorbed into the blood stream and serves to digest, or dissolve, the protein coating that protects the cancer cell from the attack of the body's white blood cells. Once this is done, the white cells move in on the cancer cells and destroy them just as if they were foreign invaders to the body. But, once again, if the pancreas is weak, or if it is "exhausted" by metabolizing too much sugar, or if the diet contains too much animal protein, then the enzyme is deficient for the job nature has cut out for it.

This is why, in our view, cancer probably should be identified as a deficiency disease. It is a disease caused by a deficiency of vitamin B_{17}, pancreatic enzymes, or both.

The foregoing is not intended as a comprehensive explanation of Dr. Krebs' theory, and much has been omitted or oversimplified for this introduction to the subject. To cover the ground adequately would take several volumes and, obviously, is beyond the scope of this book. I urge every reader interested in the scientific aspect of the Laetrile mechanism, however, to read *World Without Cancer; The Story of Vitamin* B_{17} by G. Edward Griffin[1]. It is a masterpiece of research and clarity and should be in the library of every serious student of this subject.

As mentioned previously, I soon became convinced on the basis of *theory* that the nitrilosides, consisting of amygdalin, Laetrile, and prunasin, together with the pancreatic enzyme trypsin, constituted a natural barrier against the growth of cancer. The next logical step was to confirm the theory through actual practice.

At the time I was only vaguely aware of the so-called California Anti-Quackery law. I knew that, somehow, worthless cures were prohibited by statutes, but I never dreamed how much latitude was allowed administrative public servants to define what was and what was not worthless; and never in my wildest imagination did I suspect that a multibillion-dollar drug industry had such influence over regulatory agencies of government as to constitute a virtual blockade against the development of drugless medicine.

At any rate, I was certain that none of these laws affected me. I had been licensed under Section 2146 of the California Business and Professional Code which reads as follows:

> Nothing in this chapter shall be construed so as to discriminate against any particular school of medicine or surgery, school of podiatry, or any other treatment, nor shall it regulate, prohibit or apply to any kind of treatment by prayer, or interfere in any way with the practice of religion.

This statute obviously authorized me to use *any* method of treatment, regardless of the school of medical thought behind it. Besides, there are well-estab-

---

[1]American Media, PO Box 4646, Westlake Village, CA 91359.

lished procedures for matters of this kind. If the state or the medical society learns of a practice which it considers to be illegal or unethical, it gathers information, contacts the physician in writing or in person advising him of the possibility that his actions are in question, and invites him to discuss the matter and to explain or defend his position. Then, if it is decided by the authorities that the practice in question is improper, the physician is advised again in writing and given a choice of conforming to the decision or appealing to a higher authority. It is the way things are done in a profession of honorable men. So I had little reason to suspect what was in store for me when I ordered my first small supply of amygdalin.

The first patient to receive amygdalin was Mildred Seybold, the sister of Charlotte Anderson, one of my nurses. She had an advanced malignant melanoma of the left arm. Her attending physician told her that, in his opinion, she had about six weeks to live. On the outside chance that they could slow down the process a little, he had recommended immediate amputation of the arm.

Amygdalin was administered, and almost immediately the lesions began to heal. Within two months, her arm had returned to normal appearance and function, and we put her on a maintenance oral dosage. That was the summer of 1971. The woman is alive and well today—except for the fact that, when she reduces her maintenance dosage of amygdalin, hairs begin to form on the old site and her arm begins to swell. These symptoms retreat, however, with the return to the recommended level of vitamin B_{17}. (Incidentally, this woman, who also is a diabetic, received an unexpected bonus from our therapy. When she adopted the recommended vegetarian diet, she found that she could discontinue the use of insulin and still control her diabetes.)

When Mrs. Seybold returned to her original physician for a routine check-up months later, he was dumbfounded at the fact that they could find no cancer. Yet he still wanted to amputate her arm. She asked if he would recommend that if he had never seen her before. He said no, but because he previously had seen the cancer he felt that amputation was the only safe and sensible course of action. Needless to say, she did not follow his advice.

Any physician who deals extensively with cancer patients soon learns to recognize that certain symptoms constitute what might be called a pre-clinical syndrome. The patient has no identifiable tumor or lesion, yet he complains of feelings of impending doom, malaise, unexplained or vague pains, headaches, bowel changes, loss of appetite, loss of energy, and depression. I have learned from experience that a high percentage of those who presented a combination of these symptoms developed clinically detectable cancer soon afterward. I was curious, therefore, to see what effects amygdalin would have on such cases, so I prescribed oral vitamin B_{17} along with other vitamins and waited anxiously for the results. They were exactly as I had hoped. In almost every case, the symptoms cleared up dramatically and, to this day, I have not had any of my patients progress from the pre-clinical syndrome to fully developed cancer.

Encouraged by these early results, I began to offer amygdalin to my other cancer patients. Unfortunately, most of them were, by any standard medical classification, "terminal." We had done everything that consensus medicine said should be done, and it appeared that they were going to die anyway. They readily accepted vitamin therapy without hesitation. After all, what could they lose?

The first doses, nevertheless, were, by current standards, extremely small: usually three grams or less injected once a week. I was particularly concerned about possible side-effects, since these always are major factors in the administration of all accepted cytotoxic drugs. I half expected to see the usual reactions: loss of hair, vomiting, diarrhea, dizziness, and the like.

To my delight, none of these appeared on the

charts. In their place, patients began to report a reduction in pain, an increase of appetite, a gradual return of strength, and a marked improvement in mental outlook. As an unexpected bonus, hypertensive patients also showed a return to normal blood pressure.

Although these initial results were encouraging, most of the patients ultimately passed away from the irreparable damage already done to their vital organs before therapy began. I resolved to increase the dosage level and to learn more about the effect of diet. We gradually increased the injections to six grams of amygdalin several times a week and put the patient on a strict vegetarian diet—no animal protein of any kind.[1] There was considerable grumbling about the diet, but the results told us immediately that we were on the right track. For the first time in my entire medical career, I began to see "terminal" cancer patients abandon their stretchers and wheelchairs and return to normal lives of health and vigor.

It was inevitable that word of what we were doing would get around quickly. Our office soon was filled with faces we had never seen before—hopeful faces of men and women who had been abandoned by orthodox medicine as hopeless or "terminal" cases. They came to us as a last resort for miracles, but we had none to offer. What we did provide, however, was a release from pain, a return of human dignity, a modest extension of life, and a vast upgrading of quality of that life while it lasted. Had this been the result of the orthodox therapies I had used in the past, I would have considered it immensely successful. But now, with a vision of a better way, I was not satisfied.

I continued to study and to improvise. Gradually, we increased the doses to nine grams six times per week. We added tests to determine the patient's general mineral balance, and began to stress the importance of *all* vitamins and minerals, not just vitamin B_{17}, as part of the total natural mechanism. Our

---

[1]See *appendix* for the diet recommended to our patients.

view of the patient's condition was expanded to include not just one or two malfunctioning systems but the interaction and balance of his entire body metabolism. For that reason, we began to refer to this holistic approach as "metabolic therapy."

No longer were we treating the lump or bump, we were treating the entire patient. While the medical profession continued to think of cancer as a *tumor,* we recognized it as a systemic *condition.* A lump or bump is merely the *symptom,* not the disease itself. No wonder we doctors had failed to control cancer all these years. We had been attacking the symptom and ignoring the disease.

Let's talk about those tumors for a moment. Most of them are a mixture of cancer cells and non-cancer cells. It comes as a surprise for many to learn that, in the average tumor, the greater portion of the tissue is non-cancerous. No one fully understands the mechanisms involved, but it would seem that the tumor actually is part of the body's defenses *against* cancer. When cancer begins to form, and if the vitamin and pancreatic factors are insufficient to check it, the body begins to surround it with millions of non-cancerous cells in an apparent effort to seal it off and isolate it. In a sense, therefore, the tumor really is our "friend" because it is attempting to protect us from having its cancerous content spread to other parts of the body.

In the early 1950's, tuberculosis generally was incurable and almost always fatal. The treatment of choice at that time included radical surgery to remove the Ghon tubercle, along with the lung itself. Today, such radical surgery is quite rare, and most TB sanitariums have been closed due to lack of patients. The TB "lump" no longer is viewed as something that must be removed at all costs. In fact we know that it effectively encases the live tubercle bacilli and acts as a barrier against their spread. If we were to cut into the lump or "zap" it with radiation to shrink it in size, chances are we would succeed only in destroying the natural barrier and spreading the disease.

The point is that in cancer, as in tuberculosis, our primary concern should not be whether there is a lump or bump, but whether that lump or bump is life-threatening. In most cases it is not. Consequently, at the clinic we have learned to view the tumor primarily as a cosmetic problem. If its presence is of phychological concern to the patient, we usually recommend surgical removal, but only *after* we are certain that the cancerous cells throughout the body have been minimized by metabolic therapy. Of course, if the tumor *is* threatening the life of the patient through pressure on a vital organ, such as the brain or bowel, then corrective surgery definitely is justified, and we are forced to take our chances at causing metastasis to other parts of the body as the lesser of two evils—a stop-gap measure to buy time for metabolic therapy to have a chance.

Our critics, of course, say this is quackery. They see the tumor grow, watch the patient die, and conclude that the tumor *is* the disease. That is like observing a wet sidewalk in a rainstorm and concluding that wet sidewalks either cause ran or *are* rain. It is like looking at inflation, with its accompanying rising prices, and then concluding that rising prices either cause or *are* inflation.[1] It is equally absurd in medicine to look at a tumor and conclude that it is the total cancer. Yet, that is the fundamental error that now holds back orthodox medicine and which, in fact, even is written into the California law against cancer quackery. This law decrees that cancer is a space-occupying lesion and that any therapy that does not attack that lesion is, by definition, "quackery." It decrees that unless tumor size is reduced (and reduced quickly), the therapy being used is "worthless." Moreover, it decrees that anyone who does not conform to these opinions is subject to criminal prosecution.

---

[1]Inflation, of course, is the expansion of the money supply at a rate greater than the expansion of available goods and services. Rising prices are the *result* of inflation, neither its cause nor its essence.

Section 1075 of the California Health and Safety Code defines cancer as follows: "For the purposes of this chapter 'cancer' means all malignant neoplasms regardless of the tissue of origin." According to *Taber's Cyclopedic Medical Dictionary, Twelfth Edition,* a neoplasm is defined as "a new and abnormal formation of tissue, as a tumor or growth." On page 57 of the report to the Legislature by the California Cancer Advisory Council entitled "Cancer, Cancer Quackery and Cancer Law," we find the following *Criteria for Response to Therapy:*

> In the evaluation of anti-tumor effect, only objective decrease in the size of measurable lesions . . . can be accepted as demonstrating antitumor effects by thc compound under study. Subjective effects such as pain relief, increased appetite, weight gain, increased activities . . . are not evidence of anti-cancer effect.

As long as this sophomoric attitude is accepted by orthodox medicine, and especially as long as it is forced on the rest of us by the effect of law, tens of thousands of people will continue to die needlessly *every single day,* and all the million-dollar grants and all the research in the world will fail to stop it.

What a price we pay when scientific error becomes enshrined by law.

My practice underwent a rapid transformation, and I found myself swept along somewhat helplessly by the consequences of my discoveries. I continued to administer to the needs of my old patients, of course, but word of my successes with cancer patients—spread by the patients themselves—brought far more new patients than I could handle alone. I increased the staff, tore out my X-ray machine to make more room for patient care, and soon my little neighborhood practice was converted into a busy cancer clinic with patients from many states.

The inevitable finally happened at ten in the morning June 2, 1972. Without warning of any kind, two police cars and two unmarked government cars screeched to a halt at strategic points around our clinic. Uniformed officers surrounded the building and, *with guns drawn,* nine men and one police matron burst through the front door, flashed a search warrant at the receptionist, and pushed their way on through the clinic itself. I was thrust against a wall and frisked for a concealed weapon. The nurses were confined to their station, and the patients, with one exception, were told to go home.

I was informed by the inspector from the California Health Department, that I was under arrest for violating the California "anti-quackery" law, and that his warrant authorized a search for any and all Laetrile as well as literature pertaining to it. By this time, agents were everywhere: looking in cupboards, pulling out drawers, checking the content of closets, even examining the books in my medical library to see if there were any hollowed-out secret compartments.

I refused to answer any questions until I had called my attorney. I was denied that *right!* I then asked for permission to call my wife. That, too, was denied. (Later, when my wife tried to reach me by phone, she was told I could not speak with her.) There being no alternative, I sat in silence as they rummaged through every drawer and shelf at the clinic.

They found no Laetrile, although several vials sat right out in the open. They just didn't recognize it when they saw it.

Soon after arrival, the inspector confiscated my car keys and instructed one of the officers to get my briefcase out of the trunk and take it for evidence. Incredible! For him to know that I kept all of my most important papers pertaining to Laetrile in a briefcase in the trunk of my car, he must have been watching my every move for quite awhile. The image of being spied upon from nearby windows and parked autos sent a creeping sensation down my spine.

At the time of the raid, a little girl about seven years old by the name of Kerry Alderson was in examination room number three. She had just begun metabolic therapy for an advanced case of osteogenic sarcoma (cancer of the bone). When she first came to the clinic I didn't think she had much of a chance because of the late start—and I told that to her parents. But I was willing to do everything I could for her if that is what they wanted—which it was.

Kerry had responded beautifully in terms of increased appetite, weight gain, freedom from pain, and a feeling of well-being, but her leg continued to fester and swell. In fact, as she lay on the examining table, her leg did not present a very pretty picture. The inspector took one look at it, turned pale.

Normally, Kerry would have received a massive injection of vitamins, including vitamin B_{17}. Under the circumstances, however, not being sure what kind of legal trouble I would be in if I administered amygdalin right in front of a state Health Department official who already was searching for evidence against me, I simply cleaned and dressed her lesions and sent her home. It was evident, however, that the little girl—as well as her parents—were greatly upset by the threatening presence of police officers.

The child died three days later, and there is no doubt in my mind that this death could have been postponed or possibly avoided altogether if it hadn't been for the raid which (1) interrupted the only therapy that had a chance to save her life, and (2) caused great mental and emotional trauma to the patient, which only could have diminished her resistance to the disease. I record this event here because I look forward to the day when the government can expect to be held accountable for its official acts for only on that day will the individual citizen be secure in his Constitutional liberties.

When I completed my work on Kerry's leg and sent her home, the inspector informed me that he was taking me to jail. Along with my two nurses, I was marched out the front door past TV cameramen and put into a police car.

Oh, yes, the cameramen.

They were there almost from the start. Along with police officers, they had complete freedom to wander around the clinic taking pictures and recording conversations. The whole thing was obviously rigged to do as much damage to me as possible. The press had been invited by the inspector to cover the raid. As far as the general public is concerned, when they see someone on TV being taken away by the police, *that person must be a criminal!* Regardless of who was right or wrong, the man in the handcuffs is guilty of something or they wouldn't have arrested him! It's called trial by TV, and it is a highly effective weapon in the FDA's "arsenal of compliance." If they can't get a conviction against a person in court, at least they can ruin his reputation, his business, or his medical practice by adverse publicity. The end result is the same either way.

The inspector had encouraged me to speak to the press, but I declined. If he wouldn't allow me to speak to either my wife or my attorney, I certainly wasn't going to let him push me into speaking with the press!

I was taken to the Albany jail and booked like a common criminal—and so were my nurses. I was put into a room and left alone to think.

I was in jail! I couldn't believe it. Had I really committed a crime? Yes, by definition of the California "anti-quackery" law, I had. But was there not a *higher* law that, by *its* definition, would make the California statute a crime? Surely the Constitution was such a law, and there was the California Business and Professional Code that specifically guaranteed that the state has no right to interfere in the private practice of a duly licensed physician. Also there was my Hippocratic Oath—and my moral obligation just as a human being to do what I could to alleviate pain and suffering. All of these were higher laws than some obscure statute written by lawyers, passed by politicians, and interpreted by power-mad bureaucrats. *They* were the criminals. *They* were the ones who should be sitting in cells!

Four hours after the arrest, I finally was released. I didn't know what I was going to do next, but I did know that I had just begun to fight.

II

Self-Evident Absurdities—And Other Orthodox Clichés

by John A. Richardson, M.D.

Answers to the following charges: that Laetrile is an overly simplistic approach, that the FDA would gladly test it if it held any promise, that it has not been proven safe, and that all favorable results can be attributed to delayed reaction of previous orthodox therapy or to spontaneous remission. Includes a discussion of favorable results reported by doctors from Indonesia and Israel.

A little over seventy years ago, writing in the *Journal of the American Medical Association,* Dr. Robert Reyburn and Dr. Roswell Park expressed the opinion that if the cancer rate continued to increase, "there will be more deaths from cancer than from consumption [tuberculosis], smallpox, and typhoid fever combined."[1]

From the perspective of the present day, that seems like an understatement, indeed. Yet, if we had lived at the time it was written, we would have had to depend on the experts for advice on what to believe. The most expert expert around in those days was a fellow by the name of Fredrick L. Hoffman, who wrote a book entitled *The Mortality from Cancer throughout the World.* Among Mr. Hoffman's many impressive credentials, we note that he was Chairman of the Committee on Statistics of the American Cancer Society (then called the American Society for the Control of Cancer), a member of the American Asso-

---

[1]*JAMA,* November 10, 1906.

ciation for Cancer Research, an Associate Fellow of the American Medical Association, an Associate Member of the American Academy of Medicine, etc., etc. From this there is no doubt that he was not only an expert but also a recognized spokesman for orthodox medicine.

In his book Mr. Hoffman quoted the prediction that cancer would some day result in more deaths than tuberculosis, small pox, and typhoid fever combined, and then declared: "This statement on its face is a self-evident absurdity."[1]

Very little has changed since then except the date. Spokesmen for orthodox medicine—and particularly for the American Cancer Society—continue to cloak themselves in the mantle of their own prestige, deride any scientific opinion that differs from their own, and categorically denounce as absurd those things which they do not understand. Laetrile is the current victim of such scientific arrogance and ignorance.

The orthodox medical establishment has a large bag filled with ready-made clichés to counteract any and all evidence in favor of Laetrile. To the average person, who knows nothing of the background, they can be extremely convincing. I think it is important, therefore, to take a close look at some of the most common of them.

Since we who are proponents of Laetrile view cancer as a deficiency condition, we see all kinds of cancer as merely different manifestations of a single disease process. Spokesmen for orthodox medicine reply that this is a "self-evident absurdity" because of the large variety of cancer types. To believe that there could be just one treatment for all of them is, in their view, "an overly simplistic solution to a highly complex problem."

Admittedly, there are many manifestations of the disease. According to one widely-used reference, *Cinical Oncology:*

---

[1]Hoffman, *The Mortality from Cancer throughout the World* (the Prudential Press, Newark, New Jersey, 1915), p. 41.

> More than 270 types of human neoplasms have been recognized and defined histologically, and the degrees of variation within a single tumor type can be infinite.[1]

The argument, thus, is that a single treatment for 270 types plus infinite variations of cancer is simplistic. But, first of all, no Laetrile clinician would ever advocate Laetrile without also prescribing pancreatic enzyme supplements, other vitamins and minerals, and a low animal-protein diet. So it is not exactly a single treatment. Nevertheless, let us lump it all together for the sake of comparison and *call* it one: metabolic therapy. By contrast, orthodox medicine has three treatments to offer: surgery, radiation, and chemotherapy. Is that really significantly less simplistic? If so, then perhaps we should have 270 treatments to do the job right. But what, then, of the "infinite" variations.

Experience has proven that the greatest gains in medicine have been made not through complexity but simplicity. All the conquered diseases of man have been beaten by a single substance, a single therapy, based upon a single *proper* understanding of the disease itself. As long as orthodox medicine is unable to demonstrate what the cause of cancer *is,* its spokesmen would be well advised to become more humble about labeling the theories of others, especially when those theories have the weight of medical experience on their side.

Another common cliché used against Laetrile is that, if there is any value in it, its developers should obtain a permit from the FDA to test it under scientifically controlled conditions and publish their results so the medical community can properly evaluate it. The implications in this are that (1) the developers never have tried to obtain an FDA permit and (2)

---

[1]*Clinical Oncology for Medical Students and Physicians.* Third Edition, 1970-1971, (The American Cancer Society in conjunction with the University of Rochester School of Medicine, Rochester, N.Y.), p. 20.

they are not willing to reveal the results of an honest, scientifically controlled experiment.

Here are the facts. The McNaughton Foundation applied to the FDA for permission to test Laetrile on April 6, 1970. Permission was granted on April 27. The very next day, the FDA drafted a letter stating that extensive additional data would be required *within ten days,* or the permit would be rescinded. The letter arrived on May 6, leaving the McNaughton Foundation only two days to prepare literally hundreds of additional pages of data. The permit was cancelled on May 12.

Andrew McNaughton proceeded with the paperwork anyway, believing that the permit would be reinstated upon its completion. The job was finished on May 15 and everything that had been requested was sent off to Washington. The FDA, however, has steadfastly refused to grant the permit to test.

One of the reasons given for refusing is that Laetrile might be toxic. They said: "It is dangerous to initiate human studies while the nature of the toxicity has not been elucidated in large animal species."[1]

To anyone with any knowledge of the subject at all, that is an incredible statement. Amygdalin has been well-known and listed in the *United States Pharmacopeia* as a non-toxic substance for over a hundred years. The human case studies submitted by McNaughton were further proof of its safety. To deny permission to test on the grounds that amygdalin *may* be toxic is mind-boggling when one realizes that virtually all drugs currently approved by the FDA for cancer therapy are *extremely toxic.*

Even without these considerations, one is faced with the fact that the amount of red tape now required for clearance of a new drug by the FDA is so great and so expensive that only the very largest drug companies can afford to comply. This fact has led many observers to conclude that the red tape actually

---

[1]The Ad Hoc Committee of Oncology Consultants for Review and Evaluation of Amygdalin (Laetrile), FDA, Aug. 12, 1971, pp. 3, 4.

was created specifically to serve the interests of the large firms and to squeeze out competition from smaller firms which can afford neither the paperwork nor the political lobbying required to gain favoritism.

In 1948, Parke, Davis & Co. was able to get a license for a new drug after submitting seventy-three pages of information. In 1968, the same company was required to submit 72,200 pages of data to accomplish the same purpose. One drug company had to present 456 volumes of data, weighing one and a half *tons,* to secure a license for a simple muscle relaxant.[1] It is widely accepted that if penicillin, insulin, or even aspirin were submitted for clearance today, they could never make it through the FDA maze of requirements and paperwork.

Prior to the enactment of the FDA's present new drug standards, an average of 41.5 "new chemical entities" came on the market each year. In the years following, the average dropped to only 16.1. University of Chicago economist Sam Peltzman estimates that a two-year delay in introducing drugs to combat tuberculosis—which would be a minimum at present—would have resulted in 45,000 additional deaths from that disease.

There are no patents on vitamin B_{17}. If one did have five million dollars to spend on complying with the FDA's preapproval requirements, there would be no way to recover it, since every drug and vitamin firm in the world could manufacture it freely. In my opinion that the current FDA red tape is condemning innocent people to death, and I feel the government's refusal to allow Laetrile to be used experimentally is nothing less than genocide.

As mentioned previously, no one with real knowledge of the subject claims that amygdalin is toxic. Yet, apparently more to frighten the public away from Laetrile than anything else, spokesmen for orthodox medicine never tire of hinting at the possibility that people will be poisoned if they eat foods rich in vitamin B_{17}.

---

[1] "The Medicine Man," *Private Practice,* May, 1975, p. 49.

There have been repeated scare articles about one or two people who allegedly became ill after eating apricot kernels, but none of them could ever be verified. The latest salvo from that gun battery is an article in the *Journal of the American Medical Association*[1] which discusses the alleged dangers of "chronic cyanide intoxication" as manifested in some Nigerian farmers who "subsist on cassava diets." Cassava is unusually rich in vitamin B_{17}, and the article in question uses this as one more proof of the invalidity of amygdalin as a control for cancer.

Few would question such an article appearing in a prestigious medical journal, and almost no one would bother to check it out. Yet if they did, here is what they would find. One of the world's foremost authorities in the field of chemical toxicity is Dr. O. L. Oke at the University of Ife, Ile-Ife, Nigeria. In January of 1976 he completed an unusually comprehensive study of the effects of cassava on the chemistry of the body. He showed that, while different animals have different tolerances for the cyanide component of vitamin B_{17}, actual toxicity is extremely rare for any of them. To the contrary, he pointed out that experiments with high-nitriloside foods quite frequently produced stronger and healthier animals than before the experiments began. Then he said:

> The degree of toxicity depends on the degree of hydrolysis by intestinal glucosidase to release the toxic agylcone, also when orally administered. Thus taken orally it is less "toxic" than almost any vitamin. . . .
>
> Cassava is very poor in protein and vitamins and the protein is also of poor quality. . . . This poor amount is further decreased when cassava is processed to gari or lafun. Thus gari, lafun, and purpuru all are mainly carbohydrates with hardly any proteins and hence it would not be surprising that using any of these as the sole source of diet could result in a deficiency disease.

---

[1]Sept. 13, 1976, p. 1284.

> From both animal and human evidence on the relation of neuropathies to cyanide content of food, it seems that apparent core relation between the two is an expression of the general deficiency of the diet rather than an expression of the specific effect of cyanide.[1]

The subject of cassava is a good place to introduce the next orthodox cliché, which runs something like this: "There is no evidence that Laetrile works. Don't you think that we want to find a cure for cancer just as much as anyone else? Believe me, if there were any shred of evidence that it worked, no matter how faint, we would follow up on it. But no such evidence has ever been produced." The latest in this cacophony of wide-eyed sincerity comes from Robert C. Everly, spokesman for the American Cancer Society, who put it this way:

> For twenty years, we have asked the proponents of Laetrile for scientific documentation of efficacy, but it has not been forthcoming.[2]

As reinforcement to this theme, a long list of "scientific experiments" usually is cited in which allegedly it was proven that Laetrile failed completely to produce any evidence of anti-cancer activity.

Griffin has already exposed the ineptitude of these "experiments"[3] for anyone who has the interest to pursue this sordid record of corrupted science. Let us point out in passing, however, that (1) in almost every case the "patients" tested in these experiments were mice (which do not have the same metabolism as humans), (2) the tumors were transplanted (which do not react the same as spontaneous tumors), and

---

[1] "The Prophylactic Action of Cassava," by O. L. Oke, Ph.D., University of Ife, Ile-Ife, Nigeria, transmitted Jan. 20, 1976, pp. 36, 37. (To be published in the journal of the International Society for Tropical Root Crops, Cali, Columbia.)

[2] *Ca-A Cancer Journal for Clinicians,* American Cancer Society, Jan./Feb., 1976, vol. 26, no. 1, p. 52.

[3] *World Without Cancer; the Story of Vitamin B₁₇, op. cit.,* pp. 17-46.

(3) in all of the experiments cited, *reduction of tumor size* was the primary criterion for evaluating results, and (4) there is nothing quite so easy to accomplish as failure.

As I have stated earlier, the foundation theory supporting the use of Laetrile is that the tumor is merely the symptom of the disease, that most tumors have only a relatively small proportion of cancer cells; consequently, getting rid of the cancer often leaves behind a tumor of benign tissue as a memorial to the victory of nature over the disease. To use the reduction of tumor mass as the primary test of efficacy is indefensible from a scientific point of view and is further evidence of the appalling ignorance of orthodox researchers.

It is a well-known fact that most cancer patients die, not from the tumor, but from something called *cachexia.* Cachexia is the medical term used to describe the loss of weight and appetite, a decrease of strength, the appearance of anemia, an increased basal metabolism rate resulting in a caloric and nutritional deficit, and a general "wasting away" that is seen in terminal cases. According to the New York Academy of Sciences:

> Cachexia, of course, is of major clinical significance in patients with cancer. Warren reported that cachexia was the most frequent single cause of death in cancer, especially of the stomach, breast, and colon-rectum groups. The pathogenesis of this cachexia remains unknown at present.[1]

If it is true that cancer patients die not from the tumor but from a wasting away of the body, then wouldn't we be doing the patient a favor if we could, somehow, improve his appetite, return his strength, and re-build his body weight? This, in fact, *is* one of the

[1]"The Anorexia-Cachexia Syndrome: A New Hypothesis," Athanasios Theologides, *Annals of the New York Academy of Science,* vol. 230, March 18, 1974, p. 17.

primary objectives of treatment, and a great deal of space is devoted in the medical literature to this very problem. For instance, in the physician's handbook *Current Diagnosis and Treatment,* we find the following statement:

> A valuable sign of clinical improvement is that of the general well-being of the patient. . . . Factors included in the assessment of general well-being include improved appetite and weight gain and increased performance status.[1]

With this in mind, let us turn to the pages of one of the most often cited "scientific experiments" which allegedly proved that Laetrile was worthless. It is the famous *California Report* released by the Cancer Commission of the California Medical Association. Its conclusion was stated bluntly and categorically: "No satisfactory evidence has been produced to indicate any significant cytotoxic effect of Laetrile on the cancer cell." But on page five, the report said:

> All of the physicians whose patients were reviewed spoke of increase in the sense of well-being and appetite, gain in weight, and decrease in pain *as though these observations constituted evidence of definite therapeutic effect.* [Emphasis added]

As the saying goes, "Let us reason together." If it is of primary importance that medicine find a solution to cachexia in cancer patients, why, then, at the same time scoff at the fact that those of us using Laetrile *have* found a solution? The answer, of course, is that these so-called scientific experiments all are being conducted by lump and bump doctors who haven't yet learned to look beyond the tumor to the disease itself.

But let us return to the subject of cassava. At the

---

[1](Lange Medical Publishing Co., Los Altos, California, 1972), p. 902.

Cisarua Health Resort in Bogor, Indonesia, 175 cancer patients were given a high-concentration cassava diet specifically to observe what effects, if any, it would have on their disease. A few patients did experience a slight dizziness and nausea but these were easily counteracted by standard symptomatic treatment. Dr. Simandjuntak, who helped to conduct the experiment, wrote:

> Up till now, of the ± 6,000 patients who already have been treated with SPP Cassava tuber [175 of whom were being treated for cancer], none have even shown any sign of dangerous intoxication. Detected were only faint spells of dizziness, which easily were neutralized by drinking a glass of sweet tea.[1]

The important part of this study, however, was not the lack of toxicity; it was the effect on the patient's disease. After detailing the administrative and clinical procedures used, Dr. Simandjuntak summarized his findings:

> After administration of SPP Cassava to the patients, clinical progress can be observed, e.g.
>
> 1. Improved eating/sleeping.
> 2. Reduced feelings of pain.
> 3. Feelings of being more fit.
> 4. Increased body weight.
> 5. The tumor mass becoming weaker/smaller (in some cases a total disappearance of the tumor mass was detected) . . .
>
> From the 175 carcinomas, patients' clinical progress after the administration of treatment with SPP Cassava have been detected in 67 cases, or in ± 38%. . . .
>
> The patients suffering from malignant breast tumor who came to Cisarua Health Resort in Bogor for treatment have mostly received sur-

---

[1] "A One Year Experience of Treating Breast Tumors With Sao Pedro Petro Cassava (SPP)", by Todotua Simandjuntak, M.D., *Medika,* vol. 1/I, August, 1976.

gery and radiation already. . . . *The best progress through treatment with SPP Cassava was detected on patients who previously had not received any medical intervention.* [Emphasis added][1]

In the summer of 1976, a team of physicians from Israel visited the Laetrile clinics currently in operation in Mexico and the United States. When they returned, the head of the team, Dr. David Rubin, Surgeon at the Beilinson Hospital and Cancer Researcher at the Hadassah Hospital in Jerusalem, drafted their report to the Israeli Ministry of Health. Here, in part, is what it said:

SUMMARY OF OBSERVATIONS CONTAINED IN REPORT OF 1 SEPT 1976

1. With few exceptions, all of the cases we saw were advanced incurable cancer patients. Most of them had had conventional therapy before being treated with LAETRILE.

2. The most striking observable feature was relief of pain accompanied by a decrease or even cessation of the need for pain killers and sleeping potions. It is interesting to note that in the majority of cases the patients came off long-term use of narcotics without the usual withdrawal symptoms.

3. After a few days of treatment with LAETRILE there was an improvement in appetite followed, in many cases, by a gain in weight.

4. A frequent striking feature in cancer wards is the odor of decaying cancer masses. We observed that this fetor is generally absent in the cases of patients under LAETRILE therapy.

5. LAETRILE is non-toxic to normal somatic cells and may be given by injection in doses up to 5 grams per kilogram of patient weight per day. . . .

In short, it is our conclusion that:

a. Contrary to many allegations in both

---

[1]*Ibid.*

the scientific and lay literature, LAETRILE is not quackery.

b. LAETRILE is non-toxic even in very large doses.

c. LAETRILE has a definite palliative effect. We cannot, at this stage of our investigations, say that it inhibits tumors, but the evidence we have suggest that it does. We must do controlled studies to rule out the possibility that prior therapies had some effect on the tumors that stopped growing. However, we doubt that the regressions we observed were due to "delayed effects" of other therapies because, in our experience, *such delayed effects rarely, if ever, occur.* [Emphasis added][1]

There will be more to say presently on the subject of "delayed effects" of orthodox therapies but, for now, let us keep to the main subject, which is the allegation that there is no evidence to support the claims on behalf of Laetrile. As I hope you are beginning to see, the evidence is, in fact, abundant. For instance, the regions of the world where the native diet is high in nitrilosides are exactly the same regions where the people are noted for their good health, longevity, and freedom from cancer. In the United States there is a well-defined group of Laetrile advocates who consistently reinforce their daily diet with vitamin B_{17} supplements. While their fellow citizens now are suffering from cancer at the rate of one out of every four, not one of these people has ever been known to contract this disease. All of this has been presented and documented by Griffin in *World Without Cancer; the Story of Vitamin B_{17}*,[2] and the facts are well established in the scientific literature.

When finally confronted with some of the evidence that Laetrile is effective, the critics can be counted on to fall back to the next line of defense

[1]Report 2#, "Use of Laetrile in the Prevention and Treatment of Cancer", by David Rubin, M.D., Oct. 25, 1976. Copy in author's files.

[2]*Op. cit.*

and complain that the evidence is *invalid* because there has been no control group to verify that the results are not produced by psychological factors (the placebo effect) or, as mentioned in the Israeli Report, by the delayed reaction of previously administered orthodox therapies.

The thought that we should have conducted double blind studies is appalling. First of all, those of us who have been using Laetrile have been treating human beings, not guinea pigs. It would be unconscionable to give half of my patients an injection of saline solution or, for that matter, to prescribe radiology or toxic chemotherapy. In my mind I would know that I was not giving the first group the metabolic therapy they need to prolong or save their lives, and the second group I would be condemning to disfigurement, untold suffering, and almost certain death. Only those who have no faith in Laetrile could entertain the idea of a control group.

Besides, do not all the patients now dying in our nation's cancer wards constitute a sufficient control group! I gladly will put up our modest case histories against any similar number of orthodox cases, and I believe the comparison will speak for itself.

As for the placebo effect, the possibility that our patients are merely "psyching themselves up" and responding to a kind of faith healing, one can only say that, of course, we have no mesmeric powers. In fact, we go out of our way to explain to all new patients that, if the cancer is far advanced or if there has been extensive damage done by prior radiation or chemotherapy, the chances for their recovery are quite slim.

Belief in Laetrile *can* be a factor leading to a more healthy, emotional state and to a more cooperative attitude toward our therapy—both of which are important. Many of our patients, however, have no faith in Laetrile at all and come to us only to please a spouse or a relative. Yet, if they adhere to the total metabolic regimen as prescribed, their response is identical to those with unbounded faith.

It is hard to imagine how a "dumb animal" could

respond to the placebo effect, so let's look briefly at the results obtained by veterinarians. Dr. George Browne, Jr., who heads the Eureka Veterinary Hospital in Eureka, California, published a highly revealing case history in the February, 1974, issue of *Pet Practice*. The patient was a five-and-a-half-year-old male Pekingese dog with a biopsy-established diagnosis of thyroid carcinoma. Although the complete case is included in this book's appendix, the concluding paragraphs are these:

> The twice-weekly regimen was continued for one month, during which time the growth regressed to a size comparable to that palpated during the original examination. Intravenous injections were discontinued and a daily maintenance dosage of 100 mg. of amygdalin per orum was established. This dosage has been continued for seven months.
>
> A biopsy taken six and one-half months after the initiation of amygdalin therapy revealed no evidence of malignancy.[1]

In another case, Dr. Browne described a ten-year-old mixed-breed female dog that underwent surgery in 1972 to remove a tumor on the gum above the right upper canine tooth. The pathologist identified it as a squamous cell carcinoma. On January 5, 1973, the dog was referred to the Veterinary Clinic at the University of California at Davis for evaluation and possible radiation therapy. The University Clinic reported that the cancer had invaded so much of the bone as to make treatment virtually impossible. The owners were so advised and elected to keep the dog until such time as the cancer would make it sufficiently uncomfortable to warrant having it euthanatized.

After describing this background, Dr. Browne reported:

---

[1] "Remission of Canine Thyroid Carcinoma Following Nitriloside Therapy", by George Browne, Jr., D.V.M., *Pet Practice,* Feb. 1974, p. 189.

> On January 16, the owners consented to experimental treatment with amygdalin. The dog was given 1,600 mg. of amygdalin intravenously on alternate days until 12 treatments had been given. When the last two injections were given, a small amount of amygdalin solution was infiltrated directly into the visible portions of the lesion.
>
> On February 10, when intravenous treatments were discontinued, oral administration of amygdalin was started at a dose of 100 mg. daily. After seven days without development of overt side effects, the dose was increased to 400 mg. daily. . . .
>
> By November 24, the lesion appeared to be completely healed. Administration of amygdalin was continued at 400 mg. per day until January 16, 1974. The dosage was then reduced to 100 mg. per day and kept at that level. . . .
>
> The Patient has been followed, and to date [April, 1976] there has been no recurrence of the lesion.[1]

It is unlikely, to say the least, that dogs are responding to faith healing or to the placebo effect. So let us turn next to that ever-popular claim that favorable Laetrile results actually are but the delayed reaction of radiation or chemotherapy. This can become awfully convincing at first simply because the majority of our patients indeed have been exposed to such orthodox treatments long before they show up at our clinic. The fact is, however—as Dr. Simandjuntak discovered, and as all Laetrile practitioners have confirmed—the more prior radiation and chemotherapy a patient has received the *less* likely it is that he will respond to Laetrile, or anything else. As the following chapter shows quite conclusively, the customary "delayed reaction" of orthodox therapy is death.

If one were to keep count of all the patients who

---

[1]"Remissions of Canine Squamous Cell Carcinoma After Nitriloside Therapy", by George Browne, Jr., D.V.M., *Pet Practice,* Nov. 1976, p. 1561. Full report included in *appendix.*

have been classified as terminal with only a few weeks left to live, and then record the number who suddenly had favorable delayed reactions to their radiation or chemotherapy, subsequently regaining their health and vigor, there probably wouldn't be more than a hundred such cases per year in the entire United States. Yet, from my own files and those of just one or two other Laetrile practitioners, there could be assembled several thousand of such cases each year. Any serious attempt to attribute all of these favorable responses to a mechanism that is known to be so extremely rare is certainly the height of desperation.

So, as a final resort, a last-ditch effort to discredit Laetrile, especially in those cases where there has been no prior orthodox therapy for the supposed delayed reaction, the critics finally fall back to the claim that these cases represent "spontaneous regressions," that the cancer just went away on its own, not as a result of Laetrile, but as a result of a return of the natural resistance of the host.

It is true that occasionally a patient will recover from cancer without any treatment whatsoever. This fact tells us something important. It tells us that the body *does* have some kind of *natural* control for the disease, if we only knew what it was. One thing is certain, whatever it is, it is *not* X-radiation or toxic chemicals.

The statistical probability for spontaneous regressions, is just about the same as for delayed reactions. Most official estimates are 1 in 80,000 to 100,000 cases.[1] Warren Cole, Emeritus Professor of Surgery at the University of Illinois College of Medicine, reviewed the spontaneous remission cases reported in all the medical literature from 1960 to 1966. Including cases dating back to the early 1900's there were exactly 92 cases that had a survival rate of two years or more.[2]

---

[1]"Spontaneous Regression of Cancer: The Metabolic Triumph of the Host?" *Annals of the New York Academy of Science,* Vol. 230, *op. cit.,* pp. 111, 112.
[2]*Ibid.,* p. 112.

If these really are cases of spontaneous remission, then it should be noted that I have more such cases at my own clinic than the rest of the world combined. It would seem that we get a much higher rate of "spontaneous remissions" using Laetrile than with anything else we've ever tried!

Yes, the evidence that vitamin B_{17} is nature's control for cancer is quite overwhelming. So the next time you hear an official spokesman for orthodox medicine proclaim that there is none, you might tell him that such a statement is a "self-evident absurdity" and suggest that he do his homework before posing as an expert.

And you might also remind him that, by definition, a "quack" is one who pretends to have knowledge which, in fact, he does not.

III

The Hoax of the Proven Cancer Cure; A Second Look at Orthodox Therapy

by G. Edward Griffin

Brief historical review of court decisions and legal sanctions against physicians using Laetrile; analysis of assumptions supporting the anti-Laetrile laws and administrative rulings; close look at medical results obtained from surgery, radiation, and chemotherapy, demonstrating that none of them properly can be considered a "proven cure," as claimed by the American Cancer Society and other proponents.

Mr. Griffin is author of many documentary books and films, including *World Without Cancer; the Story of Vitamin* B_{17}, and is president of American Media.

On July 21, 1967, the trial of Dr. Maurice Kowan was coming to a close. His "crime" was the use of Laetrile in the control of cancer. In a crowded courtroom in Los Angeles, prosecuting attorney Ira Reiner solemnly faced the jury and said:

> This is not a kindly old man. This is the most thoroughly evil person the imagination can concoct. He's taking advantage of people for money.
>
> We can understand people who kill in rage. What do you think of a man who can kill at nine dollars per visit? . . .
>
> This man has to be stopped. He is very dangerous. This case goes far beyond the walls of this courtroom. The way to stop him is a guilty verdict.[1]

---

[1]"Kowan Trial Nearing End in City Court," L.A. *News-Herald & Journal*, July 23, 1967.

The jury had never been allowed to see any evidence that Laetrile actually worked. They believed every word the prosecutor said. Three days later, they pronounced Dr. Kowan guilty. He was fined $4,400 and, at age 70, sentenced to two months in prison.

Dr. Kowan was not the first Laetrile proponent to feel the wrath of organized medicine. In 1956 Dr. Arthur T. Harris, who had been successfully treating cancer patients in Sherman Oaks, California, was summoned by the county medical society to attend a special meeting at *two o'clock in the morning*. He was threatened with suspension, loss of his hospital privileges, and legal prosecution. Pickets were hired to parade in front of his office warning patients that he was a quack. In utter despair, Dr. Harris closed his practice, sold his home, and became a medical missionary in South Africa.

In April of 1973, Dr. Byron Krebs was arrested and convicted for using Laetrile in the control of cancer. His brother, Dr. Ernst T. Krebs, Jr., the biochemist who first synthesized Laetrile, also was convicted of "practicing medicine without a license." They were fined $500 each and placed on three years' probation.

In November of 1975 Dr. Stewart M. Jones of Palo Alto, California, was tried by the state Board of Medical Examiners and found guilty of treating cancer patients with Laetrile. He was severely reprimanded, told that he would lose his license if he continued, and was put on a two-year probation. He was arrested five months later when state agents raided his office and found one vial and ten Laetrile tablets.

On December 16, 1975, Dr. James Privitera was convicted in a San Diego Superior Court for conspiring to use Laetrile as a control for cancer. His sentence was six months in prison and five years' probation.

On March 22, 1976, Dr. Seymour Weisman was convicted in an Arizona court on the charge of illegally transporting Laetrile. His sentence was three months in a federal prison.

Dr. John Richardson, of Albany, California, has faced perhaps more legal harassment from the state than any other physician. He has had his license suspended, has been arrested, hauled off to jail twice, and four times made to stand trial for using Laetrile. He has spent more than six months defending himself in court. In the fourth trial they succeeded in securing a conviction against him, but he has appealed his case, and the battle continues. Regardless of the outcome, the bureaucracy has unlimited resources and will not let up in its efforts either to stop him legally, to exhaust him financially, or to destroy him through adverse publicity.

To the average observer the FDA's attitude toward nutritionally oriented physicians is incomprehensible. Thousands of voices have been raised in protest, but the federal and state agencies merely reply that they are protecting the consumer from "quackery."

The laws and administrative rulings prohibiting the use of Laetrile are justified to the public (and to the juries) on the basis of two assumptions. The first is that Laetrile is completely worthless or, at best, "unproven." The case histories that constitute the main portion of this book show quite dramatically that such an assumption is incorrect. The other assumption, however, is even more important because it is the backbone of the argument in favor of such laws. It is the argument that orthodox therapies—surgery, radiation, and chemotherapy—are "proven cures" which offer the patient an excellent chance of recovery if only started in time. If this assumption is correct, as we are told it is repeatedly by spokesmen for these therapies, then the gullible public must be prevented from seeking Laetrile, not so much because it is worthless or unproven but because it prevents the patient from obtaining the truly effective and "proven" cures of orthodox medicine.

This theme is presented in the American Cancer

Society's book, *Unproven Methods of Cancer Management*. It says:

> Unfortunately, many patients with curable cancer leave the care of competent physicians to be treated with a worthless unproven remedy until a cure by accepted methods of treatment becomes impossible.[1]

Section 10400.1 of the California Health and Safety Code has embodied this sentiment into law as follows:

> . . . the use of [Laetrile] in early cancer to the exclusion of conventional treatment with acceptable modern curative methods (surgery or radiation) would thereby be delayed potentially until such time as metastasis had occurred and the cancer therefore might no longer be curable.

An American Cancer Society brochure asks the question: "Why not use an unproven method if it has been proven to be harmless?" Then it answers:

> Because time is cancer's ally. Any time wasted on worthless unproven remedies may prevent a patient from obtaining proven treatment while his cancer is still curable.

In response to this statement, a letter was sent to the American Cancer Society headquarters expressing surprise at the assertion that there was any cancer therapy successful enough to warrant being called a proven cure. This is the reply:

> Thank you for your note. There *are* proven cures *if* detected in time—surgery and/or radia-

---

[1]1971 edition, p. 1.

tion and, more and more, chemotherapy is playing a part.[1]

This, then, clearly is the position of orthodox medicine. The purpose of this chapter is to take a second look at these so-called proven cures and to demonstrate that the scientific record does not support their claim.

Surgery has been the primary treatment for cancer at least from the time of the Egyptians. Celsus, in the first century, left excellent descriptions of surgery for cancer of the lip. Leonides in the Second Century, and Guy de Chauliac in the Fourteenth Century described a wide variety of operations for cancer. Hildanus described the first axillary dissection for breast cancer in the Sixteenth Century. The first radical operation for breast cancer was described by Halstead in 1891, and his basic procedures are still followed today.

In many cases, cancer surgery can be a lifesaving, stop-gap measure—particularly where intestinal blockages and adhesions must be relieved to prevent death from secondary complications. Surgery also has the psychological advantage of visibly removing the tumor, and, from that point of view, it offers the patient and his family some temporary comfort and hope. The degree to which surgery is useful, however, is the same degree to which the tumor is *not* malignant. The greater the proportion of cancer cells in that tumor, the less likely it is that surgery will help. Generally the most highly malignant tumors of all are considered inoperable.

One of the primary problems with surgery is the fact that any cutting into the tumor—even for a biopsy—usually results in spreading the cancer to other parts of the body. This is a grim fact that most physicians fail to tell their patients when they recommend biopsy. According to *Clinical Oncology for Medical Students and Physicians* (published jointly by the University

---

[1]Letter from Mabel Burnett dated December 18, 1972.

of Rochester School of Medicine and The American Cancer Society) even massaging a tumor should be avoided. It says:

> Massage of a tumor is followed by massively increased numbers of circulating tumor cells in the blood stream. . . . Experimental data further suggest that surgical trauma decreases natural host resistance to the formation of metastasis. . . .
>
> Needle biopsy is occasionally used, [but] . . . a needle track may harbor nests of cells which may form the basis for a later recurrent spread. Incisional biopsy of certain highly malignant tumors through an open operative field may be contraindicated because of risk of spread of the tumor throughout the operative field.[1]

Writing in the *Annals of the New York Academy of Sciences,* Dr. Warren Cole spoke a truth that is well-known within the medical profession but almost completely unknown to the public at large. Speaking of a series of surgical experiments, he wrote:

> Ten of our patients underwent an unsuccessful attempt by a surgeon to remove the tumor. *All surgeons know that this procedure is usually followed by an increased growth of the tumor. . . .*
>
> Although the most common factor related to spontaneous regression in our monograph was excision [removal] of the primary [tumor], I cannot attach much importance to it because *metastasis* [spread of the cancer] *develops so commonly after excision of the primary.* [Emphasis added][2]

In view of the many problems and dangers inherent in cancer surgery, one may wonder why phy-

---

[1]*Clinical Oncology for Medical Students and Physicians, op. cit.,* pp. 32, 34.

[2]"Spontaneous Regression of Cancer: The Metabolic Triumph of the Host?," *op. cit.,* pp. 136, 137.

sicians recommend it. The expected answer, of course, is that, statistically, a patient stands a better chance for survival *with* surgery than *without* it, in spite of all the risks. The facts, however, are not that comforting. There is a growing awareness even among many of the world's top surgeons that patients who submit to surgery have no greater life expectancy, on the average, than those who do not. Let's take a look at the record.

The first statistical analysis of this question was compiled in 1844 by Dr. Leroy d'Etoilles and published by the French Academy of Science. It is, to date, the most extensive study of its kind ever to be released. Over a period of thirty years, case histories of 2,781 patients were submitted by 174 physicians. The average survival after surgery was only one year and five months—not much different than the average today. Dr. d'Etoilles separated his statistics according to whether the patient submitted to surgery or caustics, or refused such treatment. His findings were startling:

> The net value of surgery or caustics was, in prolonging life, two months for men and six months for women. But that was only in the first few years after the initial diagnosis. After that period, those who had not accepted treatment had the greater survival potential by about fifty per cent.[1]

Of course 1844 was a long time ago. But recent surveys invariably have produced nearly the same results. For instance, it long has been accepted practice for patients with breast cancer to have, not only the tumor removed, but the entire breast and the lymph nodes as well. In more recent years, the procedure often includes subsequent removal of the ovaries also.

---

[1]Walshe, Walter H., *The Anatomy, Physiology, Pathology and Treatment of Cancer*, (Ticknor & Co., Boston, 1844).

In 1961, a large-scale controlled study was begun to see if all the extra surgery was worthwhile. It was called the National Adjuvant Breast Project. After seven and one-half years of statistical analysis, the results were conclusive: there was *no* significant difference in the percentage of patients remaining alive between those who had received the smaller operations and those who had received the larger.[1] These findings were well publicized in medical literature in 1969. Yet, even today, radical breast surgery continues to be performed in every hospital in America—fully approved by consensus medicine.

Cancer statistics can be very misleading, as we shall discuss shortly. Nevertheless, let us see what they tell us about survival possibilities after surgery. Two of the most common forms of cancer leading to surgery are of the breast and the lung. According to current medical literature, only sixteen per cent of those undergoing breast surgery will experience a long-term survival. In the case of cancer of the liver it is twelve per cent; with lung cancer it is ten per cent; of the pancreas it is four per cent.[2] As low as these figures seem, they actually are quite high when compared to survival expectations for some of the less common cancer locations.

When we turn to cancers which have metastasized to secondary locations within the body, then the odds drop practically to zero—surgery or no sur-

---

[1]Ravdin, R. G., *et al.*, "Results of a Clinical Trial Concerning the Worth of Prophylactic Oophorectomy for Breast Carcinoma, *Surgery, Gynecology and Obstetrics,*" 131:1055, Dec. 1970. Also see "Breast Cancer Excision Less with Selection," *Medical Tribune,* Oct. 6, 1971, p. 1.

[2]See "Results of Treatment of Carcinoma of the Breast Based on Pathological Staging," by F. R. C. Johnstone, M.D., *Calif. Medical Digest,* Aug., 1972. Also "Consultant's Comment," by George Crile, Jr., M.D., *Surgery, Gynecology & Obstetrics,* 134:211, 1972, p. 839. Also, "Project Aims at Better Lung Cancer Survival," *Medical Tribune,* Oct. 20, 1971. Also statement by Dr. Lewis A. Leone, Director of Oncology at Rhode Is. Hosp. in Providence, as quoted in "Cancer Controls Still Unsuccessful," L.A. *Herald Examiner,* June 6, 1972, p. C-12.

gery. As Dr. Johnstone summarized it in the pages of *California Medical Digest:*

> A patient who has clinically detectable metastases when first seen has virtually a hopeless prognosis, as do patients who were apparently free of distant metastasis at that time but who subsequently return with distant metastasis.[1]

An objective appraisal, therefore, is that the statistical rate of long-term survival after surgery is, on the average, *at best* only ten or fifteen per cent. And once the cancer has metastisized to a second location, surgery has almost *no* survival value whatsoever. The reason, of course, is that, like the other therapies of orthodox medicine, surgery removed only the tumor. It does not remove the cause.

The first reported use of X-rays in the treatment of cancer was in 1899. The first radium brought to the United States was given to the New York Academy of Medicine in 1903. The development of machines such as the cobalt and proton accelerators are comparatively recent, but the rationale behind them all is essentially the same as with surgery. The medical objective is to remove the tumor, but to do so by burning it away rather than cutting it out.

The average tumor is a mixture of cancer and non-cancer cells. The grim fact of radio therapy is that normal cells usually are more easily damaged by X-rays than cancer cells. The result is that the tumor reduces in size by giving up its non-cancer component. The portion that remains may be smaller, but its concentration of malignancy is greater.

Dr. John Richardson has explained the phenomenon this way:

> Radiation and/or radiomimetic poisons will reduce palpable, gross or measurable tumefac-

---

[1]Johnstone, *op. cit.*, p. 838.

> tion. Often this reduction may amount to seventy-five per cent or more of the mass of the growth.
>
> For example, a benign uterine myoma will usually melt away under radiation like snow in the sun. If there be neoplastic cells in such tumor, these will remain. The size of the tumor may thus be decreased by ninety per cent while the relative concentration of definitively neoplastic cells is thereby increased by ninety per cent.
>
> As all experienced clinicians know—or at least should know—after radiation or chemotherapy have reduced the gross tumefaction of the lesion, the patient's general well-being does not substantially improve. To the contrary, there is often an explosive or fulminating increase in the biological malignancy of his lesion. This is marked by the appearance of diffuse metastasis and a rapid deterioration in general vitality followed shortly by death.[1]

And so we see that X-ray therapy is cursed with all the same limitations and drawbacks of surgery—including the fact that it actually increases the likelihood that cancer will develop in other parts of the body!

Yes, it is a well-established fact that excessive exposure to radioactivity is an effective way to induce cancer. *The Encyclopaedia Britannica* says:

> Energy from the ultraviolet rays of sunlight, and ionizing radiations from X-ray, radium, and other radioactive materials encountered in industry and in the general environment cause a variety of cancers. The pioneer workers with radium and X-rays developed cancers of the skin. Even now, radiologists and others exposed to high total doses of ionizing radiation are more likely to develop leukemia than persons not so exposed. Uranium miners have been found to have a higher than normal incidence of lung cancer.[2]

---

[1]Open letter to interested doctors, Nov., 1972.
[2]Fifteenth edition, p. 764,

The *Textbook of Medical-Surgical Nursing,* a standard reference for registered nurses, is most emphatic on this point. It says:

> This is an area of public health concern because it may involve large numbers of people who may be exposed to low levels of radiation over a long period of time. The classic example is of the women employed in the early 1920's to paint watch and clock dials with luminizing (radium-containing) paints. Years later, bone sarcomas resulted from the carcinogenic effect of the radium. Similarly, leukemia occurs more frequently in radiologists than other physicians. Another example is the Hiroshima survivors who have shown the effects of low levels of radiation. . . .
>
> Among the most serious of the late consequences of irradiation damage is the increased susceptibility to malignant metaplasia and the development of cancer at sites of earlier irradiation. Evidence cited in support of this relationship refers to the increased incidence of carcinoma of skin, bone, and lung after latent periods of 20 years and longer following irradiation of those sites. Further support has been adduced from the relatively high incidence of carcinoma of the thyroid 7 years and longer following low-dosage irradiation of the thymus in childhood, and from the increased incidence of leukemia following total body irradiation at any age.[1]

In 1971 a research team at the University of Buffalo, under the direction of Dr. Robert W. Gibson, reported that fewer than a dozen routine medical X-rays to the same part of the body increase the risk of leukemia by at least sixty per cent.[2] Other scientists have been increasingly concerned about the growing

---

[1](J. B. Lippincott Co., Philadelphia, PA., 1970) 2d Ed., p. 198.
[2]"Too Many X-rays Increase Risk of Leukemia, Study Indicates," *National Enquirer,* Dec. 5, 1971, p. 11.

American infatuation with X-rays and have urged a stop to the madness, even calling for an end to the mobile chest X-ray units for the detection of TB.[1] Dr. Erwin Bross, director of biostatistics at the Roswell Park Memorial Institute of Cancer Research, has called for an immediate stop to the nation-wide X-ray screening program for the detection of breast cancer. He charged that the American Cancer Society and the National Cancer Institute had ignored the objections of scientists and had rammed through the program so they could receive government grants totaling fifty-four million dollars to carry out the screening. Dr. Bross warned that the program caused far more cancer than it detects. He said:

> For each woman who is possibly cured by early detection, there are four or five new cancers produced by these X-rays. . . . In my view this entire matter has become so serious that the NCI would be better off putting the money allotted for future screenings into a trust fund for the victims of the program who will develop cancer in ten to fifteen years' time.[2]

It is important to bear in mind that these routine, diagnostic X-rays are harmlessly mild when compared to the intense "therapeutic" radiation beamed into the bodies of cancer patients.

Since X-rays *cause* cancer, not *cure* it, it is not surprising that X-ray therapy has a statistically high rate of failure. The National Surgical Adjuvant Breast Project, previously mentioned in connection with sur-

---

[1]"Top FDA Officials Warn: Chest X-Rays in Mobile Vans Are Dangerous and Must Be Stopped," *National Enquirer*, Sept. 10, 1972, p. 8. Also *Textbook of Medical-Surgical Nursing, op. cit.* p. 199.

[2]"Expert Blasts Two Cancer Groups that Pushed Breast X-Ray Program," *National Enquirer*, Nov. 30, 1976, p. 49. Also "Breast Cancer: Looking for A Cure Becomes A Cause," *Mother Jones*, Nov. 1976, p. 6.

gery, also conducted studies on the effect of irradiation, and here is a summary of the findings:

> From the data available it would seem that the use of post-operative irradiation has provided no discernible advantage to patients so treated in terms of increasing the proportion who were free of disease for as long as five years.[1]

There are many adverse side effects of X-ray therapy. Anyone who has witnessed the grotesque disfigurement of a patient's face—the loss of a nose or a jaw with the remnant covered with hideous scar tissue—will not soon forget it. It is common for internal adhesions or destruction of nerve muscles to leave the patient hopelessly crippled and, of course, in pain. The patient's white blood cell count drops, resulting in a susceptibility to infections and other diseases.[2] A simple cold can lead to death from pneumonia. As Dr. Richardson expressed it, "It's the cobalt that will kill, not the cancer."

For obvious reasons, radiologists seldom publicly discuss their high failure rate. If they did, there soon would be few patients coming to their doors willing to undergo the pain and disfigurement. To learn the truth, therefore, one has to go to the professional journals where radiologists speak to their own fraternity. Here are just a few examples. Dr. William Powers, Director of the Division of Radiation Therapy at the Washington University School of Medicine, has stated:

> Although preoperative and postoperative radiation therapy have been used extensively and for decades, it is still not possible to prove un-

---

[1]Fisher, E., *et al.* "Postoperative Radiotherapy and the Treatment of Breast Cancer; Results of the NSABP Clinical Trial," *Annals of Surgery,* 172, No. 4, Oct. 1970.

[2]"Impaired Immunoresponsiveness in Tumor Patients," by Jules Harris, M.D., and David Copeland, M.D., *Annals of the New York Academy of Sciences,* Vol. 230, March 18, 1974, p. 56.

equivocal clinical benefit from this combined treatment.[1]

Dr. Phillip Rubin, Chief of the Division of Radiotherapy at the University of Rochester Medical School, says:

> The clinical evidence and statistical data in numerous reviews are cited to illustrate that no increase in survival has been achieved by the addition of irradiation.[2]

Dr. Vera Peters, radiologist at the Princess Margaret Hospital in Toronto, Canada, states:

> . . . There has been no true improvement in the successful treatment of the disease over the past thirty years.[3]

And from the pages of the *American Journal of Roentgenology,* we find this:

> In many quarters the superiority of combination therapy is accepted as established dogma, and re-examination of treatment policies viewed as heretical. Despite the confident air of this position, a life-sparing effect specifically attributable to the radiotherapeutic component of combination regimens has not been proven.[4]

---

[1]"Preoperative and Postoperative Radiation Therapy for Cancer," speech delivered to Sixth National Cancer Conference, sponsored by the American Cancer Society and the National Cancer Institute, Denver, Colorado, Sept. 18-20, 1968.
[2]"The Controversial Status of Radiation Therapy in Lung Cancer," speech delivered to the Sixth National Cancer Conference, sponsored by the American Cancer Society and the National Cancer Institute, Denver, Colorado, Sept. 18-20, 1968.
[3]"Radiation Therapy in the Management of Breast Cancer," speech delivered to the Sixth National Cancer Conference, *op. cit.*
[4]"The Role of Postoperative Irradiation and the Management of Stage I Adenocarcinoma of the Endometrium," by C. Paul Morrow, Philip J. Di Saia, and Duane E. Townsend, *American Journal of Roentgenology,* Aug. 1976, p. 325.

In view of these facts, it is tragic to contemplate the number of human beings who have been scarred, disfigured, and crippled for life by a therapy which, according to its own practitioners, is *"unproven."* If anti-quackery laws are indeed written to protect the public from unproven cures, then we look forward to the time when the American Cancer Society will launch a public crusade against radiology, and when the FDA will put a padlock on all radiology machines, and when those who now claim that radiation is a cure for cancer are made to stand trial for medical quackery.

Let us turn now to the third "proven cure" of orthodox medicine: *chemotherapy*—treatment by drugs.

The first use of drugs in cancer therapy occurred in 1919 when nitrogen mustard was used in an effort to control leukemia. The theory behind almost all chemotherapeutic drugs introduced since then has been the same. Generally they are strong poisons that are given to the patient in the hope that the cancer cells in his body will die before he does.

That is not an exaggeration. The chemicals are selected because they are capable of differentiating between types of cells and, consequently, of poisoning some types more than others. Unfortunately they can *not* distinguish between cancer and non-cancer cells. Instead they differentiate between cells that are fast-growing and those that are slow. Cells that actively are dividing are the targets. Consequently they kill not only cancer cells that are dividing but also a multitude of normal cells all over the body that happen to be caught in the act of dividing.

In the case of those cancers that are dividing more rapidly than normal cells, theoretically they will be killed before the patient is. In the case of a cancer that is dividing at the *same* rate or slower than normal cells, then there isn't even a *theoretical* chance of success.

In any event, the poisoning of the system is the whole objective of these drugs, and the resulting pain and illness often is a torment worse than the disease itself. The toxins catch the blood cells in the process of dividing and cause blood poisoning. The gastrointestinal system is thrown into convulsion causing violent nausea, diarrhea, loss of appetite, cramps, and progressive weakness. Hair cells are fast growing, so usually the hair falls out during treatment. Reproductive organs are affected, causing impotency or sterility. The brain becomes fatigued and wracked with pain. Eyesight and hearing are impaired. In fact, every conceivable function is disrupted with such agony for the patient that many elect to die of the cancer rather than continue treatment.

It is a well established fact that one of the body's best defenses against cancer is a healthy and well-functioning immunological system—the white blood cells. As stated in the *Annals of the New York Academy of sciences:*

> The importance of the immune system in the defense against neoplastic disease [cancer] seems established. The high incidence of cancer of various types in patients with immune deficiency diseases and in patients who have received immunosuppressive therapy, especially after kidney transplantation, supports the concept that rejection of an incipient malignancy is an important function of the immune system . . .[1]

Recently, there has been increasing evidence that oncogenesis [the creation of new cancer cells] is not an unusual event but that, instead, most cancers are destroyed by the immune system before they develop into a clinically recognizable disease.[2]

Dr. Warren Cole, Emeritus Professor of Surgery

---

[1]Vol. 230, *op. cit.*, p. 45.

[2]"Current Knowledge and Concepts of the Relationships of Malignancy, Autoimmunity, and Immunological Disease," by George J. Friou, M.D., *Annals of the New York Academy of Sciences,* Vol. 230, March 18, 1974, pp. 44, 45, 48.

at the University of Illinois College of Medicine, has said that even in cases where cancer *has* developed into a clinically recognizable disease the natural resistance of the body is still the most important medical consideraiton—more important than the tumor itself.[1]

With this in mind, we return to the chemotherapeutic drugs currently accepted by orthodox medicine, and we discover that almost all of them produce, as a side-effect, *the destruction of the patient's immunological defense mechanism!*[2]

It should be obvious that if one of the body's main defenses against cancer is knocked out by chemotherapy, then chemotherapy will *produce* more cancer than it *cures*—which is exactly what the record reveals.

The first evidence to this effect was a marked increase in lung cancer among those who worked on the manufacture of mustard gas during World War II.[3] Then it was observed that kidney transplant patients who were given these same immunosuppressant drugs developed cancer at fifty times the normal rate.[4] A recent experiment conducted for the National Cancer Institute showed that all of the currently accepted drugs in the American Cancer Society's "proven cure" category produced cancer in laboratory animals that previously had been healthy![2] And, yet another study at the National Cancer Institute showed that those patients who underwent intensive chemotherapy developed secondary cancer at a rate 270% greater than those who did not.[5]

---

[1] "Spontaneous Regression of Cancer: The Metabolic Triumph of the Host?" *op. cit.*, p. 130.

[2] "Impaired Immunoresponsiveness in Tumor Patients," *op. cit.*, pp. 56, 67, 72.

[3] *The Encyclopaedia Britanica,* Fifteenth edition, vol. 3, p 764.

[4] NCI research contract PH-43-68-998.

[5] "Recently Recognized Complications of Cancer Chemotherapy," by James C. Arseneau, *et. al., Annals of the New York Academy of Sciences,* Vol. 230, March 18, 1974, p. 485.

Dr. Dean Burk, while head of the Cytochemistry Division of the National Cancer Institute, made the following observation in a letter to the head of the NCI. He said:

> Virtually all of the chemotherapeutic anti-cancer agents now approved by the Food and Drug Administration for use or testing in human cancer patients are (1) highly or variously *toxic* at applied dosages; (2) markedly immunosuppressive, that is, destructive of the patient's native resistance to a variety of diseases including cancer; and (3) carcinogenic [cancer-causing]. . . . I submit that a program and series of the FDA-approved compounds that yield only 5-10% "effectiveness" can scarcely be described as "excellent," the more so since it represents the total production of a thirty-year effort on the part of all of us in the cancer therapy field![1]

Dr. Saul Rosenberg, Associate Professor of Medicine and Radiology at Stanford University School of Medicine, has said:

> Worthwhile palliation [temporary relief of symptoms] is achieved in many patients. However, there will be the inevitable relapse of the malignant lymphoma, and, either because of drug resistance or drug intolerance, the disease will recur, requiring modifications of the chemotherapy program and eventually failure to control the disease process.[2]

The *Textbook of Medical-Surgical Nursing* says bluntly: "As yet no drugs are available to cure most malignant tumors."[3] Dr. Robert Sullivan at the Lahey

---

[1]Letter dated April 20, 1973, copy in author's files.

[2]"The Indications for Chemotherapy in the Lymphomas," Sixth National Cancer Conference proceedings, *op. cit.*

[3]*Op. cit.* p. 874.

Clinic Foundation says: "No chemical agent capable of inducing a general curative effect on disseminated forms of cancer has yet been developed."[1] And the *Annals of the New York Academy of Sciences* says: "A cure from chemotherapeutic agents is not considered valid."[2] And yet, in spite of this clear scientific record of failure, spokesmen for orthodox medicine continue to assure the unsuspecting public that chemotherapy indeed is one of the "proven cures."

Dr. James D. Watson, Nobel Prize-winner in medicine for his work on the structure of the DNA molecule, has said:

> The American public is being sold a nasty bill of goods about cancer. While they're being told about cancer cures, the cure rate has improved only about one per cent. The grim cancer statistics are about as bad as ever. Today, the press releases coming out of the National Cancer Institute have all the honesty of the Pentagon's.[3]

Six hundred and fifty thousand new cases of cancer are reported each year in the United States. At the present time, about one million Americans are undergoing one or a combination of orthodox treatments for cancer. The figures tell us that almost half of them will die before the year is out. Eighty-five per cent of them will be dead within five years.[4] And of those with

---

[1]Speech made at the National Cancer Institute Clinical Center Auditorium, May 18, 1972.

[2]"Spontaneous Regression of Cancer: The Metabolic Triumph of the Host?" *op. cit.*, p. 130.

[3]As quoted by attorney George Kell in testimony before the California Assembly Committee of Health, May 20, 1976.

[4]*Textbook of Medical-Surgical Nursing, op. cit.*, p. 873. Also, statement to the press at White House conference by Dr. Frank J. Rauscher, head of NCI, dated May 5, 1972. Also, refer to statement by Dr. Charles Moertal of the Mayo Clinic quoted by Griffin in *World Without Cancer; The Story of Vitamin* B_{17} (American Media, Westlake Village, Calif., 1974) p. 203. Note that published statistics of American Cancer Society are far more optimistic than this due to factors to be explained presently.

distant metastasis, only one per cent—one out of a hundred—will survive.[1]

One of the most prominent statisticians in the medical field is Hardin B. Jones, Ph.D., professor of medical physics and physiology at the University of California at Berkeley. As a recognized authority on cancer demography, he was invited to address the 1969 conference of the American Cancer Society. He began by pointing out that there usually is a wide difference between the published statistics, which indicate a *high* success rate, and the actual results of practicing physicians who universally experience a *low* success rate. He explained that this was due to several factors which resulted in statistical bias and error.

One such error arises due to the fact that the tabulations increasingly have been loaded with easy-to-control skin cancers (which previously had gone unreported) plus a large number of conditions which may not have been cancer at all. He said:

> Beginning in 1940, through redefinition of terms, various questionable grades of malignancy were classed as cancer. After that date, the proportion of "cancer" cures having "normal" life expectancy increased rapidly, corresponding to the fraction of questionable diagnosis included.[2]

Private Practice magazine for physicians touched upon this subject in its May, 1975, issue. It quoted a prominent cancer statistician who said: "I wouldn't be surprised if they're 'curing' a lot of leukemia that never existed."[3]

We are reminded that one of the side-effects of

---

[1]*The Encyclopaedia Britannica,* Fifteenth edition, Vol. 3, p. 766.
[2]"A Report on Cancer," paper delivered to the ACS 11th Annual Science Writers Conference, New Orleans, Mar. 7, 1969.
[3]"Cancer: Now the Bad News," by Daniel S. Greenberg, *Private Practice,* May, 1975, p. 67.

X-ray therapy and chemotherapy is the suppression or near-destruction of the patient's immunological defenses against infections and other diseases. A simple cold often leads to death from pneumonia—and *that* is what appears on the death certificate, not cancer. If these people properly were counted as cancer deaths, the statistics would tell quite a different story.

Back at the American Cancer Society conference, Dr. Jones turned his attention to a survival comparison between those patients who underwent orthodox therapy and those who accepted no treatments whatsoever. He pointed out that the published statistics are extremely unreliable on this score because they unfairly favor the "treated" category. He said:

> All reported studies pick up cases at the time of origin of the disease and follow them to death or end of the study interval. If persons in the untreated or central group die *at any time* in the study interval, they are reported as deaths in the control group. In the treated group, however, deaths which occur before completion of the treatment are rejected from the data, since these patients do not then meet the criteria established by definition of the term "treated." The longer it takes for completion of the treatment, as in multiple step therapy, for example, the worse the error. . . .
>
> In the comparisons it has been assumed that the treated and untreated cases are independent of each other. In fact, that assumption is incorrect. Initially, all cases are untreated. With a passage of time, some receive treatment, and the likelihood of treatment increases with the length of time since origin of the disease. Thus, those cases in which the neoplastic process progresses slowly are more likey to become "treated" cases. For the same reason, however, those individuals are likely to enjoy longer survival, whether treated or not. Life tables truly representative of untreated cancer patients must be adjusted for the fact that the inherently longer-

lived cases are more likely to be transferred to the "treated" category than to remain in the "untreated until death."

The apparent life expectancy of untreated cases of cancer after such adjustment in the table seems to be greater than that of the treated cases. [Emphasis added.]

One must remember that Dr. Jones was speaking at an official national conference of the American Cancer Society, an organization that annually produces tons of literature containing exactly the kind of erroneous statistics he was describing. He knew that what he was saying would not be popular, so he stated his conclusions as gently as possible to soften the blow. Several years later, however, he was interviewed by the press and spoke more bluntly:

> You see, it is not the cancer that kills the victim. It's the breakdown of the defense mechanism that eventually brings death. With every cancer patient who keeps in excellent physical shape and boosts his health to build up his natural resistance, there's a high chance that the body will find its own defense against the cancer. He may have many good years left in good health. He shouldn't squander them by being made into a hopeless invalid through radical medical intervention which has zero chance of extending his life.[1]

If it is true that orthodox therapies do not control cancer, then why is "early detection" so important? The answer? It isn't. In fact, it's just the opposite. The sooner orthodox therapies begin, the sooner the patient is exposed to life-destructive forces that will decrease his chances for survival.

According to the *British Medical Journal*, statistical evidence to support the value of early detection

---

[1]As quoted in *Midnight*, Sept. 1, 1975.

can be obtained only through what it calls "rigid selection of biologically favorable cases."[1] And this is not difficult to do. The large cancer clinics usually accept only those patients which, in their opinion, have the best chance of survival. So only the best biologically selected cases end up in their statistics. As one specialist told *Private Practice* magazine: "Clinical researchers don't like to treat dying patients, and poor risks can be sent elsewhere to die."[2]

Dr. Jones summarized the point this way:

> It is utter nonsense to claim that catching cancer symptoms early enough will increase the patient's chances of survival. Not one medical scientist or study has proven that in any way. . . .
>
> My studies have proved conclusively that *untreated cancer victims actually live up to four times longer thant treated individuals.* [Emphasis added.[3]

This, then, is the status of orthodox cancer therapy. Surgery is valuable primarily as a stop-gap measure and often spreads the disease to other parts of the body. Radiology weakens the patient's natural resistance to all diseases, including cancer, and actually causes cancer in otherwise healthy individuals. Radiologists admit bluntly that the value of their therapy has *not* been proven. Chemotherapy is even worse and often kills the patient before the cancer does. And, when the errors are stripped out of the published statistics, we find that those who receive no treatment at all live up to four times longer than those who accept these so-called proven cures.

The statistics that follow are taken from the National Cancer Institute, the American Cancer Society,

---

[1]"Curability of Breast Cancer," *British Medical Journal,* Feb. 21, 1976, p. 414.

[2]"Cancer: Now the Bad News," *op. cit.* p. 68.

[3]*Ibid.*

and from the clinical records of those physicians who have used Laetrile in the treatment of their own patients. They vary widely depending on the age of the patient, the sex, the cancer location, and the degree of malignancy. Consequently, the figures shown will be averages for *all* kinds and *all* groups together. This is the story they tell:

Of those with advanced, metastasized cancer, who have been told by their physician that there is no hope, only fifteen per cent will be saved when they turn to vitamin therapy—which is not good. But under orthodox treatment, less than one out of one thousand, or one-tenth of one per cent, will survive five years.

Of those with early-diagnosed cancer, at least eighty per cent will be saved by vitamin therapy. But no more than fifteen per cent will survive under orthodox treatment.

And of those who presently are healthy with no clinical cancer to begin with, close to one hundred per cent can expect to be free from cancer as long as they routinely obtain adequate amounts of vitamin B_{17}. But those who subsist on the typical American diet and rely only on the therapies of orthodox medicine are doomed to a survival rate of just eighty-four per cent. And that figure includes all ages. It is much less for those above thirty.

As mentioned previously, these figures will vary widely depending on age, sex, cancer location, and degree of malignancy. Also, they are somewhat arbitrary when it comes to separating early-diagnosed cancers from those that are advanced, for often there is a gray area between the two. Nevertheless, in general, they are as accurate as any such tabulation *can* be, and they tell an impressive story that cannot be brushed aside.[1]

We have spent billions of dollars and millions of

---

[1]For the analysis of the meaning, limitations, and sources of these tabulations, see chapter XI of *World Without Cancer; The Story of Vitamin B_{17}*, by Griffin *op. cit.*

man hours on the War on Cancer. The result is depicted clearly in the cancer death rate. In 1900 it was 62.9 per thousand. In 1905 it was 71.4. In 1910 it had grown to 76.2 In 1913 it was 78.9. In 1933 it jumped to 105. In 1948 it was 143. In 1960 it rose to 155.1. In 1976 it was 171.[1]

We have had surgery literally since the year one; radiation since the late 1800's; chemotherapy since 1943; and still the cancer death rate goes up each year. It is obvious that orthodox medicine does *not* have the answer.

The "proven cures" of the American Cancer Society do not exist. In view of the record, they are an affront to our intelligence, and they constitute one of the most tragic myths of the Twentieth Century. Undoubtedly they are useful for fund-raising purposes but they cannot be supported by the scientific record.

This myth is one of the assumptions used to justify government action against those who wish to use Laetrile. It is one of the assumptions that has caused respected physicians—whose only crime is that perhaps they are ahead of their time—to be subjected to legal harassment, ruinous publicity, professional sanctions, fines, and actual imprisonment.

The assumptions are wrong. The laws based upon those assumptions are wrong also, and the time for a change is now.

All scientific progress is tempered by the fire of controversy. Throughout history, every new idea has been met by the fierce resistance of the *status quo*. The emerging scientific truth always has prevailed, ultimately, but if the force of government was used against

---

[1]These rates are taken from death tables published by the American Cancer Society and the National Cancer Institute. Where a discrepancy exists between the two, an average figure is needed. Some may find fault with using statistics from organizations which are herein condemned as unreliable sources. We have used them, however, because (1) statistics are not available elsewhere, and (2) if they are in error, they probably conceal a *worse* picture and, thus, make our case even stronger.

CANCER DEATH RATE PER 100,000 POPULATION IN THE UNITED STATES

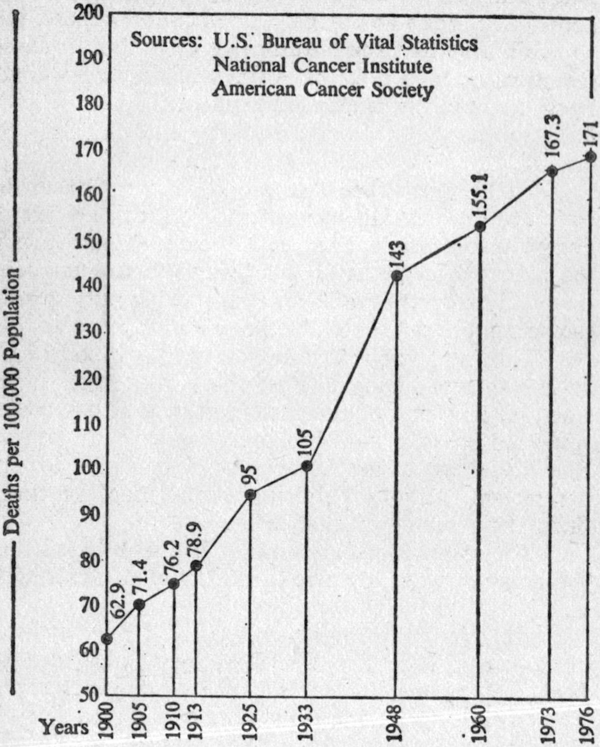

CANCER *DEATH RATE,* AS OPPOSED TO INCIDENCE, IS A REFLECTION ON THE SUCCESS OF MEDICAL PRACTICE. THE *DEATH RATE* FROM CANCER HAS NEARLY TRIPLED SINCE 1900. This chart includes patients treated with surgery, radiation, and chemotherapy, and those few people who received no treatment. (The 1976 figure was a "projected" estimate obtained from one of the above sources.)

it, it often was held back, temporarily condemned as heresy and denied recognition for centuries to follow.

We cannot afford such nonsense in the field of cancer. The lives of 360,000 Americans are at stake every year. So we simply cannot let any one side in the controversy have an exclusive medical monopoly. Unless and until the experts can come up with a lot better results than they now have, they should get off the backs of those who seek a different way.

IV

A Constitutional Scenario

by John A. Richardson, M.D.

The history of the state's early attempts to force me to stop using Laetrile, with particular attention to the unethical tactics used; my decision to be my own lawyer; the logic behind my Constitutional defense.

After my release following the first arrest, I went home and spent the evening in a state of semishock. Before the week was over, I came to learn firsthand the tremendous power of TV and the press. My acquaintances, neighbors, and even many of my patients had begun to keep their distance and now were viewing me with a mixture of caution and distrust. After all, I *had* been arrested.

The scenario that I was supposed to follow after such public humiliation and legal jeopardy was (1) to take a month-long vacation to lick my wounds, (2) to promise the authorities never to use Laetrile again, and (3) perhaps move to another part of the country and take a salaried position as an examining physician in some state or county hospital.

It didn't work out that way. Immediately after my arrest; a group of personal friends and several of my patients came together to formulate plans for my defense. They organized several hundred supporters almost immediately, and these wonderful people appeared *en masse* at the preliminary hearings leading up to my trial. Their support was extremely gratifying and served to strengthen my determination to stand on principle, even if I had to go to prison for what I knew to be right.

The pre-trial hearings, depositions, interrogatories, and conferences were numerous and dragged on for several months. Naturally, the crowds dwindled with the passage of time, but my determination did not.

Just before Christmas, a "slow plea" hearing was arranged between my attorney and the judge. It lasted about fifteen minutes. The two men exchanged legal phrases and code words of their fraternity as if sprinkling a magic potion on the victim of some voodoo curse. And then it was all over. I didn't understand any of it except that supposedly it all had been "worked out" so that I wouldn't go to prison.

One week later I was notified that I had been found guilty of something and that I had to appear before the judge for sentencing!

I was flabbergasted and angry. I did not consider myself to be a criminal, and I was not going to accept a guilty verdict without a fair trial—even if that had been part of the deal to obtain a suspended sentence. I would rather go to prison defending the truth than obtain freedom at the price of compromise with error and falsehood. I resolved to go against the advice of my attorney and stand on principle.

Fortunately I had not waived my right to a jury, so the verdict was appealed on that basis and a trial date set.

The trial itself was long, tedious, and expensive. For four weeks the prosecution presented witness after witness to create in the jury's mind the impression that I was an unscrupulous quack responsible for the agony and death of untold legions. These, presumably, would have been restored to health and happiness if only they had never come under my evil care nor been subjected to my worthless nostrums. My membership in the John Birch Society was brought up on several occasions, with heavy innuendoes that this revealed in me a fanatic suspicion of the motives of government agencies and government officials. (In this, of course, the prosecutor was absolutely correct. If I hadn't been suspicious previously, that particular government official's performance in court—his distortion of the facts, his total disregard for the truth—soon would have made me so.)

Fortunately most of the jury didn't buy it. The verdict was seven to five in favor of "not guilty."

Naive as I was, I was jubilant. "I had won!" I thought. "Now they'll leave me alone, and I can go back to practicing medicine."

My joy was short-lived. Several days later I learned that the state had decided to re-try the case, and I found myself starting all over again with pre-trial hearings and conferences leading up to what was destined to become another grueling four-week trial.

It suddenly became quite clear. They not only were trying to get a conviction against me, they also were trying to bankrupt me. Before the end of that third trial, I was destined to spend about $60,000 and the legal expenses continued to roll in. But at that point in time, I could see no alternative. Back into court I went, with attorney fees piling up at the rate of $100 per hour.

The trial was almost a carbon copy of the previous one with one exception: the jury. As we were to learn later, there were several members of the jury who appeared to be personally interested in convincing the others to find me guilty. Juror Lela Herbert told us later that she was offered financial help for her decorator shop if only she would change her vote to "guilty." Between shouting insults and threats, on the one hand, and offers of money, on the other, they literally had her in tears. Several of the others ultimately changed their votes under similar pressure, but she stood firm and would not compromise her convictions. The final vote was eleven to one.

Unable to secure a unanimous verdict, the prosecution called for yet another trial, but the judge ruled against it on the basis that justice would not be served. He said that the state had failed three times to get a conviction and that a fourth trial would be a waste of taxpayers' money. It was a narrow victory. But it was still a victory and I felt that this surely was the end.

It was just the beginning.

It was difficult for me at first to believe that a government official, especially one who was responsible for prosecuting those who violate the laws, would resort to or tolerate tampering with a jury. But I had much to learn. For instance, in April of 1976, during the trial of Dr. Stewart Jones of Palo Alto, California, an undercover agent for the state Department of Food and Drug testified that she had been ordered by James Eddington, head of the Berkeley fraud division, to make false statements in her report in order to obtain the arrest and conviction of Dr. Jones for using Laetrile. When Natasha Benton arrived in court to give her testimony, friends of Dr. Jones overheard her arguing in the hallway with Mr. Eddington and Deputy District Attorney Michael Popolizio. Miss Benton was insisting that she would not get on the witness stand and perjure herself but would tell the truth. As a result, Popolizio and Eddington decided not to call her to testify. Whereupon defense attorney David Gill *did* call her to testify, and here is the pertinent part of her remarks taken directly from the official court transcript:

> MISS BENTON: Before any report is always written, Mr. Eddington left instructions what for [*sic*] me to write. After I read these instructions, I telephoned Mr. Eddington telling him I didn't feel all those instructions were correct. He told me, "Go ahead and write what I said, because this is what we need to get a conviction." I wrote as close to what he said as I could, according to my conscience. But I still don't feel that I told the truth in that report. Later, on June 1st, I was shown a quite lengthy report. He told me to sign that report before I went before the Grand Jury, and I could read it later; we didn't have time at that time.
>
> ATTORNEY GILL: Did you sign that report without reading it?
>
> MISS BENTON: Yes, I did. Later I read a small

> portion of it. That isn't the report I wrote. Outside of this courtroom he admitted that it isn't the report I wrote. He said my report—quote—was so shitty, that that's why he changed it—close quote. . . . Mr. Eddington did ask me . . . specifically to put that Dr. Jones said it [Laetrile] was a cancer cure.[1]

This was the same James Eddington who approached my patients and their families attempting to persuade them to sue me for malpractice. He knew that any physician is bound to have a few unhappy patients or disgruntled relatives of patients, particularly when most of his cases involve terminal cancer, as mine did at that time. Eddington knew also that such suits would look very convincing to a jury, so he approached my patients with an offer of assistance if they would only agree to lend their names. Most of them refused and told us about it afterward. Two of them, however, became convinced by Eddington that it was their duty as law-abiding citizens to cooperate, so they did.

One of them, Mr. Kapitan Zema, had initially responded quite well to our metabolic therapy but, when his tumor failed to shrink in size, he became alarmed and returned to orthodox treatments.

The other individual was the father of Dorothy Soroka, who had been telling his daughter all along that Laetrile was quackery. This case never materialized however because Dorothy staunchly defended the quality of her therapy and, much to the consternation of Mr. Eddington, continued to improve. In a personal letter to me she stated:

> The treatment which I received at your office this year was taken entirely voluntarily by me. I was satisfied with it.
>
> You did not state that the treatment would cure my cancer at any time. I understood that its main purpose was to help me nutritionally.

---

[1]Transcript of proceedings, pp. 43, 44, 46.

Perhaps the most damaging device to come out of the government's "dirty tricks" department is the charge, widely circulated in the press, that I had deposited over two-and-one-half-million dollars into various bank accounts in the years 1973 and 1974. The obvious implication was that I must be making a killing out of Laetrile. Also the government was playing on the fact that many Americans are suspicious or resentful of anyone with large capital resources. In the mind of some jurors there is bound to be the thought: "He's rich. He's a doctor. Rich people and doctors, too, are arrogant. They *deserve* to be humbled. I'm going to see to it that he is."

The fact of the matter is that we did deposit over two-and-one-half-million dollars into two checking accounts in the years 1973 and 1974. But what the prosecutor did not tell the jury or the public is that well over half of that money was counted twice, and some of it three times. In other words, for business reasons, we withdrew large amounts from one checking account and deposited them into another "Vitamin Purchases" checking account. Each time the money was transferred into the second account, the government counted it as *additional* money.[1]

Then there is the fact that our clinic has become a rather large operation employing four doctors (including myself), four nurses, and twelve other staff members. It costs a great deal of money just to open our doors each morning. Our telephone bill alone averages over $10,000 per year. It is not uncommon, and certainly not reprehensible, for a business of this magnitude to handle over a million dollars annually. But, as any businessman knows, to *handle* a million does not

---

[1]During the San Diego "smuggling" trial, in 1977, the Assistant U.S. District Attorney, Herbert Hoffman, followed this ploy and attempted to create the impression in the jury's mind that our gross receipts represented total profit. Acting as my own defense attorney, I was able to show the dishonesty of such an assertion, causing Mr. Hoffman a great deal of embarrassment. When the jury realized that the prosecutor was resorting to "dirty tricks," they began to be more skeptical about all that he said.

insure that one *keeps* a million. To deposit a million into one's checking account means nothing until one knows how much one writes in checks out of that account to pay the bills. The prosecutor knows all of this, but he does not mention our expenses to the jury or to the press. The result is public outrage against "quacks who are profiteering from human suffering."

While on the subject of profits, spokesmen for the American Cancer Society have told the press that I charge $50.00 or more for an injection of amygdalin, but that the same material actually can be produced for pennies! That, of course, is a lie. The *current* wholesale cost of amygdalin to our clinic ranges from $6.25 to $7.50 per vial, duty paid, from either Germany or Mexico. The vials are labelled at three grams each, but our assays indicate only about two-and-one-quarter grams, which means that our cost is approximately $3.00 per gram. The wholesale cost of domestically produced amygdalin if $5.00 per gram.[1] The average injection contains six to nine grams of amygdalin. Our cost, therefore, is between $18.00 and $45.00 per injection, depending on the source of the material and the number of grams administered. When one adds to that the fact that the price to the patient also must include the cost of the injectionist's time, office overhead —to say nothing of the doctor's fee—our average charge of $5.50 per gram is reasonable indeed; especially when compared to the cytotoxic drugs now so popular with practitioners of orthodox medicine. The average cost to our patients for the entire course of therapy at our clinic is around $2,500. In contrast, the average cost of surgery, radiation, and chemotherapy, separately or in combination with treatments, is $30,000. Even if our patients did not respond any better than those under orthodox therapy (which they most assuredly do), it is clear just where the profiteering lies.

Although all of the legal action against me up to the second hung-jury verdict had been instigated by

---

[1]*Drug Topics Red Book, 1976* (Medical Economics Co., Oradell, N.J.), p. 68.

the state of California, I was well aware that the federal Food and Drug Administration actually was the driving force and the guiding light behind it all. On June 14, 1974, the federal FDA sent an eight-page memorandum on the subject of Laetrile to all state and local health agencies. Its stated purpose was to update these agencies regarding the status of the FDA's continuing investigations and to request cooperation from them in gathering information which could be of help in building a case against Laetrile proponents. Under the heading "FDA POLICY AND APPROACH RELATING TO LAETRILE," it explained that one of the "important elements of FDA policy" includes:

> *Encouraging local medical licensing authorities to investigate and take appropriate action to deal with the use of Laetrile by physicians in their medical practice.*[1]

The memorandum then explained that "initiating regulatory action" was another important weapon in the FDA arsenal of compliance. And so it was clear that, even though the state of California appeared to have been knocked out of the picture for awhile, the federal government now would come in and pick up the crusade against Laetrile.

It didn't take long. In February of 1975 United States marshals in Minnesota, Alabama, Washington, Wisconsin, and Oregon seized shipments of Laetrile to patients who had come to our clinic and who since had returned to their homes to continue therapy on a maintenance level. I knew then that the primary purpose for such seizures was to prove that my shipments had crossed state lines, which, theoretically, put me into interstate commerce and, thus, under the regulatory authority of the federal government. I soon learned, however, that there was another purpose behind this

---

[1]Memorandum on FDA stationery, signed by Robert A. Tucker on behalf of Glenn W. Kilpatrick, Director, Division of Federal-State Relations, p. 6.

action as well. It was to mire me in a tar pit of legal requirements.

From each state where Laetrile had been seized, I received subpoenas to appear *in those states* to defend myself against a laundry list of charges for alleged crimes. It was required that I retain a separate attorney in each state, that I travel to each for trial, and that I participate in endless hearings and interrogatories. It was a lawyer's paradise but, for me, a nightmare. I couldn't afford it either in money or time. I was, after all, only one man against the forces of the federal government and the state governments combined. They literally have highrise office buildings filled with lawyers and agents living at taxpayers' expense. Money and time are no object to them.

At about this same time, the IRS moved into my office and began poring over my books, determined to find errors and discrepancies. We had paid heavily for our 1971-72 audit previously. Now a completely arbitrary and unjust assessment of $19,000 was made against me for 1973, without benefit of audit. I contested this, and the IRS agreed before appropriate witnesses that I could place the questioned sum in escrow pending a tax court hearing. My position was vindicated a year later when, after a thorough review, I actually received an $1,800 *refund* for *over*payment of 1973 taxes. In the meantime, however, the special agent from the IRS Collection Division ignored our prior agreement and became determined to deliver the killing blow. I was threatened with a lien against my home and I had come to within just ten days of the date on which it was to be issued.

The federal noose was tightening, and for the first time I began to think that I had been beaten.

Then I met John "L" Marthaler. A former insurance man, Marthaler had become interested in our income tax laws and discovered to his satisfaction that they were completely un-Constitutional. He also came to the conclusion that the legal profession, by creating a situation where only certified ABA lawyers could appear in a court to offer "counsel" to another person, had established a closed shop in the field of law, constituting a giant fraud and conspiracy against the common man. John "L", as he is known, calls the shots as he sees them. Normally that is an excellent trait but, when it results in telling the officials of the IRS to their faces that they are lying, it can lead to disastrous consequences. At any rate, he soon became a special target of IRS wrath and subsequently lost almost everything he owned. The IRS "hit" against him, his defense, and his ultimate victory in a federal jury trial was truly an epoch of individual courage.

When I first met him, I sensed the temperament of an enraged, wounded bear. I recognized it because it represented my own state of mind at that time. Others recoiled from his seeming fanaticism. I drew strength from it. John "L" had learned much from his early failures, and for several years had been helping individuals to represent themselves in court *without the expense of an attorney*. His students were winning their battles where others had lost. His entire strategy was based upon the Constitution and the criminal laws that protect it.

When we first met, his eyes locked steadily on mine, and he said: "I know all about your case, Doctor. I've been following it closely. If you want, I can help you."

A drowning man will grasp at anything that floats, and those words were the most buoyant objects I had encountered in months. I immediately made Marthaler my non-lawyer counsel and planned to face the rest of the battle, not with lawyers' weapons of procedure, technicalities, administrative determinations, case law, and compromise, but solely with the armor and sword of the Constitution.

This was my new scenario: Article One, Sections Eight and Ten of the Constitution clearly say that only gold and silver are authorized as legal tender, or money, in the United States. That provision never has been amended, so it still stands as the highest law of the land.

Every official of the federal and state government

has taken an oath to uphold the Constitution. That includes the provision that only gold and silver shall be used as legal tender. When a government official knowingly participates in any activity that acknowledges something other than gold or silver as legal tender, he has violated his oath of office. All of the government officials who have brought charges against me knowingly have participated in the collection of taxes, import duties, fines, fees, and myriad other activities involving the use of Federal Reserve notes (our current fiat paper dollars) as legal tender. Federal Reserve notes are not gold or silver. Federal Reserve notes are not backed by gold or silver, so they do not *represent* those precious metals. Therefore, all of these officials have violated their oaths of office. As such, by definition, they are guilty of perjury, which is punishable by law (Title 18, Section 1621) calling for a fine of up to $2,000, or imprisonment for up to five years, or both. A perjured public servant is a criminal, and criminals are not qualified to represent the government in court or to conduct the prosecution against a sovereign citizen.

When my friends heard of my new approach, some of them were convinced that I had gone mad. They told me it would not work. My reply was, "Perhaps not. But I *know* the other course won't work. Besides, no one has really *tried* a Constitutional defense."

The average person, secure in his home and livelihood, never having felt the crushing attack of literally hundreds of tax-supported lawyers, unthreatened by a prison sentence for merely doing what he knows is right, such a person simply cannot understand the logic of a wounded bear.

My first chance to try a Constitutional defense came on December 2, 1975. I had been summoned to appear at an interrogatory meeting by Henry I. Froshin, Assistant U.S. Attorney for the Northern District of Alabama. Also present was Paul Ragan, an FDA lawyer representing the state of Washington; Jay Geller, an FDA lawyer representing Oregon (although based in Los Angeles); and W. Sherwood Lawrence, M.D., from the California Department of Health, who had attended my second and third jury trials for the purpose of writing pro-FDA press releases for the national media. The interrogatory was an outgrowth of my countersuit to recover the Laetrile that had been confiscated by the FDA. The purpose of this particular session clearly was to ask me a thousand questions about every conceivable topic in the hope of discovering something unfavorable to me that could be used later in court. I had sat through one just like it seven months previously and, at the insistence of my attorney, cooperated fully. The result was a hundred pages of testimony on every conceivable detail—all of which was combed through by the government for minor discrepancies or errors in my memory which could be used in court to make it appear to the jury that my story was inconsistent.

I faced these men this time with a new game plan. *They* were the criminals, not I. I was not required by the Constitution to answer their questions, so I was not going to cooperate. In fact, prior to the hearing, I had sent each of these men an affidavit asking them questions relating to their oaths of office. Specifically, I asked them if they had taken such an oath, if they were familiar with the Constitutional provision relating to gold and silver, if they were aware of the statutory punishment for any public servant who used the power of his office to deny the Constitutional rights of the sovereign citizen, and so forth.

They laughed at my crude documents but, nevertheless, didn't know what to make of them. John "L" informed me that their failure to respond to my questions was *prima facie* evidence (evidence that stands on its own merit as conclusive unless and until contrary evidence is introduced) that could be used in court to disqualify them as my prosecutors.

Here is a transcript of the key part of the hearings that followed:

RICHARDSON: You know, before we go into this, I want to mention this, because you are asking me some fairly pointed questions. I understand you're quite aware of some of the documents that I have in my possession.

FROSHIN: Excuse me, Doctor, but I'm going to insist you answer my questions and you'll have your—your counsel will have an opportunity to cross-examine you at a later time. For the purposes while I have you on direct, I'm going to insist that you just limit your answers to my questions.

RICHARDSON: Well, I'm not. . . .

FROSHIN: You need. . . .

RICHARDSON: I'm not giving you an answer. I'm asking a question myself before you interrogate me. . . . We have these documents questioning whether these gentlemen have the integrity to stand before me and ask a question pertaining to guilt or no guilt based on the unquestionable right of the sovereign citizen such as myself to determine whether or not an individual who has taken an oath to uphold the Constitution. . . . The question is does he in fact have the integrity to uphold the Constitution, or is he using money paid by the government—strike that money—sums paid by the government for the purpose of carrying out *Ultra Vires* laws that are repugnant to the Constitution. . . .

How can a criminal, a man who has shown by his action that he does not have the integrity to uphold his oath to uphold the Constitution, how can he—a criminal—ask me questions at a deposition such as this?

FROSHIN: Doctor, have you finished?

RICHARDSON: I'm asking you a question.

FROSHIN: I'll ask you, does your treatment encompass—does your practice encompass the treatment of cancer patients?

RICHARDSON: Evidently you didn't hear my question.

This sort of exchange went on for about fifteen minutes, and then, indignant and frustrated, Froshin terminated the session and went directly to secure a court order requiring that I answer his questions.

The next day in the chambers of Judge Spencer Williams I was given the option of answering the questions or withdrawing my claim for recovering the confiscated Laetrile. Under the circumstances, it seemed best to withdraw. The entire matter ended there.

It wasn't exactly a major victory, but I had tested the enemy's firepower and had survived. Under the circumstances, that was victory enough.

A similar confrontation with the IRS was even more successful. I pointed out to the District Director that I was not a tax striker. I was not refusing to pay my taxes. I merely reminded him of the Constitutional definition of legal tender and then asked him to authorize me in writing to pay my income taxes in Federal Reserve notes, not gold or silver, assuring him that I would immediately comply. That was the last we heard from the IRS.

For a while the battlefield was quiet. I hoped that the war was over, but I knew better. The next wave of attack was launched on May 28, 1976. I was scheduled to testify in Sacramento before the California Legislative Health Committee on behalf of a pending bill which would legalize Laetrile in that state. It was a very important session and a very important piece of legislation. As I approached the crowded hearing room, I was seized by several plainclothes customs agents, handcuffed, and hauled off to jail. At the same time, five police and five customs agents surrounded my clinic in Albany, roughed up several of my staff, and took Ralph Bowman, my office manager, into custody also. Our bail was set at $25,000 each! (Incredible when compared to the muggers and rapists who are released with $5,000 bail or less.)

My wife, Julie, heard about my arrest on the radio and eventually was able to locate me. She made the necessary financial arrangements so that I could put up the required bail, but, to my amazement, was told that I could not do it. They actually refused my money. I was *forced* to retain a bondsman at a cost of

$2,500. It was clear that a kick-back probably had been arranged. Although that enraged me at the time, in retrospect, it really was the least of my problems. I would gladly have exchanged such small-time local graft for the extensive national corruption that I have had to combat steadily since 1971.

Meanwhile, Ralph Bowman was taken to another jail in San Francisco. He probably would have stayed there over the long Memorial Day weekend had it not been for Janice Eby, my secretary. She literally burst in on a judge and demanded to know what they were going to do with Mr. Bowman. The judge knew nothing of the matter but, because of her insistence, checked it out. Bowman was released, but only after putting up $25,000 bond!

A few days after this arrest, I was required to travel to San Diego to be arraigned in a federal court on charges of conspiring to smuggle Laetrile and conspiring to receive smuggled Laetrile. The bail finally was reduced to "own recognizance" for both Mr. Bowman and myself.

From that date forward, I was forced to travel 1,200 miles round trip between my office in Albany and the court in San Diego on an average of once each week for over six months! On many occasions I would get there for a scheduled hearing of some kind only to be informed, "Oh, that's been postponed till next Thursday. Weren't you informed of the change?" Most of the sessions, when they did occur, were over in ten or fifteen minutes.

Having fully engaged me with a frontal attack through court action, the FDA launched an attack from the rear. In a letter to the California Board of Medical Examiners they said:

> The FDA charges that Dr. Richardson has been and is engaged in conduct prohibited by law, unfounded in science, and without medical justification. We submit that such conduct is unethical and unprofessional, particularly so when it fur-

> thers the distribution of a remedy that has no established value, the promotion of which is a fraud on the public. We call the Board's particular attention to the unresponsible and dangerous advice on the treatment of cancer in which Dr. Richardson urges patients to delay surgery and to avoid radiation treatment in favor of treatment with Laetrile. This advice, if followed, has an obvious potential for disastrous consequences.
>
> For these reasons the Food and Drug Administration respectfully urges that this Board revoke Dr. Richardson's license to practice medicine in California.[1]

The hearings before the California Board of Medical Quality Assurance were scheduled from August 3 through 11, 1976, right in the middle of my required trips to San Diego for "discovery hearings" in connection with the court action against me. *Both* proceedings—the one in San Diego as well as the one in San Francisco—were initiated by the FDA and were in compliance with their memorandum of June 14, 1974, mentioned previously.

The California Board was aware of my legal involvement in San Diego, as it was well covered in the press. Nevertheless, I notified them at the beginning of the hearings that I was unable to be present or to prepare an adequate defense because I was already totally involved in defending myself in the San Diego case.

The hearings proceeded without me. Stewart A. Judson, acting as an "Administrative Law Judge"—which, of course, is no judge at all—declared that, since no documents were received in support of my request for a continuance to a later date, my request was denied "for lack of good cause."

In all honesty, it probably wouldn't have made one

---

[1]Letter on FDA stationery, dated July 22, 1975, signed by Carl M. Leventhal, M.D., Deputy Director, for J. Richard Cront, M.D., Director, Bureau of Drugs, pp. 2, 3.

speck of difference whether I had attended this star chamber proceeding or not. The hearings were not conducted in an atmosphere of objectivity or fair play. They were like Stalin's show trials: the results had been decreed; only the process remained.

Dorothy Soroka, one of my patients mentioned previously, whose father had been pressured by James Eddington into filing a complaint against me, again became the unwilling pawn in their game. In a notarized statement she declared:

> I, Dorothy Soroka, declare: That on August 6, 1976, I was bullied into testifying, against my will, in an investigative hearing by administrative law judge, Stewart A. Judson. I did not receive a subpoena but did receive a *subpoena duces tecum.* I was informed by Stewart A. Judson that I must testify even though I had not received a subpoena.

It was clear from the attitude of Judson and the others that they were not independent men with free agency. They were acting merely as part of a larger machine we have come to know as "the establishment." They were thoroughly dependent upon the political establishment for their continued livelihood and good reputations. There was virtually no chance that any of them—even if they wanted to—would be willing to stand against the power of consensus medicine and the enforcement agencies of government to defend the rights of a recalcitrant, obstructive, nonconformist like me. The results, therefore, were predictable.

On October 28, 1976, the California Board issued its final decision and report. The main thrust of the case against me was summarized as follows:

> The conventional and medically accepted modalities in the treatment of cancer are excision of the tumor or mass, radiation therapy, chemotherapy and use of hormones, separately or in combination. . . .

> Respondent utilized Laetrile and Pangamic Acid [Vitamin B_{15}] as therapeutic agents in the treatment of cancer. Laetrile and Pangamic Acid are not recognized vitamins in human nutrition. Laetrile has no known nutritional value and is unsafe for self-medication. . . .
>
> The management of cancer patients with Laetrile, Pangamic Acid, and vitamins, as prescribed by respondent, as the sole treatment of choice by the physician, to the exclusion of the aforementioned conventional modalities is an extreme departure from the standard practice of medicine. . . .
>
> Certificate No. G-2848 of John A. Richardson, M.D., respondent above-named, is revoked.[1]

Fortunately, I had acquired the assistance of three other courageous physicians at our clinic, so the loss of my particular license—although it was a terrible psychological blow, a threat to my ability to earn a livelihood in the future, and a gross violation of my Constitutional rights—didn't prevent our clinic from treating the many patients who continued to seek our help.

Not a single doctor sat in judgment against me; it was not a real court and failed to have a judge or a jury; I was not present to defend myself or to cross-examine my accusers. Nothing about this "administrative hearing" was Constitutional. These men not only had failed to uphold the Constitution and were, thus, perjured public servants, they also had acted together to deny me my rights under the Bill of Rights of the Constitution. There is a law against that, and I decided that it was about time someone reminded these government agents that they had to obey the laws just as much as the average citizens do. I prepared a law suit against each of those participating in this un-Constitutional proceeding and sought personal damages

---

[1]Decision in the matter of the accusation against John A. Richardson, M.D., before the Board of Medical Quality Assurance, Division of Medical Quality for the State of California, Oct. 28, 1976, pp. 4, 5, 11.

against them totalling $65 million. If I am successful in this suit, the net proceeds will be donated to Laetrile research and public education programs, but I am deadly serious about pursuing the matter to the bitter end. As I have said elsewhere, our personal rights will not be secure until public officials realize that they will be held personally responsible for their acts.

V

The Principles of Nuremberg

by John A. Richardson, M.D.

A review of the records showing that there actually is no valid federal law against the use of Laetrile; an explanation of why, in the absence of such law, FDA continues legal harassment of those who use it; an appraisal of the Cancer Establishment and its vested interest in the status quo; *personal concluding observations.*

It is important to set the record straight. There is no valid federal law against the use of Laetrile. The FDA claims to have jurisdiction over Laetrile on the basis of its not having been proven to be "effective" in accordance with provisions of the Food, Drug and Cosmetic Act, as amended in 1962. This amendment, however, specifically states that any substance commonly in use before the amendment was passed does not come under its jurisdiction. This has become known as the "grandfather clause." Even the FDA's own publications concede that amygdalin was sold for treatment of cancer prior to 1962.[1] Furthermore, amygdalin has been widely in use throughout the world and has been listed in the *U.S. Pharmacopeia* for over one hundred years. In fact, its sources and properties are described at great length in the 1833 edition (!) of the *Dispensatory of the United States of America.*[2]

---

[1]cf. DHEW Publication No. (FDA) 76-3007, as quoted by Dr. Dean Burk in "Fact Sheet," December, 1976, National Health Federation *Newsletter*, January, 1977, p. 3.
[2]Gregg & Elliot, Philadelphia, 1833, pp. 76-79.

The question of whether Laetrile is a "new drug" or is "grandfathered" was the central issue in the case of Rutherford *v.* U.S. In that proceeding, the Honorable Luther Bohannon, presiding judge of the U.S. District Court in Oklahoma, granted petitioner's request to forbid the FDA from preventing his bringing a personal supply of Laetrile into the country. In a decision rendered January 4, 1977, Judge Bohannon said:

> Laetrile is not to be considered a "new drug" under the law merely because the FDA has said so, rather that said determination must be supported by substantial evidence. . . . FDA Counsel admitted that no competent administrative record had ever been developed in support of the agency's determination. . . . The Court then requested that the FDA make available to the Court the written basis for the agency's determination with regard to Laetrile, no matter how casual or unstructured its form or content might be; whereupon the Court was advised that no such rationale existed in any form. Clearly, federal agencies may not rule by fiat invoking only some unexplained application of their own expertise in defense of policy decisions they have made. . . . The agency's determination was "arbitrary, capricious," and represented an "abuse of discretion."

In June of 1975, attorney Richard Frisk contacted the U.S. Customs Office in San Francisco and asked for a list of any drugs or similar substances that were illegal to bring into the country. He asked specifically if Laetrile or amygdalin was on that list. In a sworn affidavit dated November 11, 1975, Frisk stated that he "was told by the different officials in the Customs Service Office that there was no proscribed drug or substance list, that Laetrile, or amygdalin, was not on a proscribed list, that only certain dairy products were proscribed." When he asked them to confirm that in writing, they refused.

The FDA publishes a list of chemicals and natural substances that, in its opinion, are "Generally Regarded As Safe"; hence, it is known as the GRAS list. On page 320, under the heading of Essential Oils, Oleoresins, and Natural Extractives, we find the following listing: "Bitter almond (free from prussic acid) —Prunus amygdalus Batsch, Prunus armeniaca L., or Prunus persica L. Batsch." These are almond, peach, and apricot seeds!

Dr. Dean Burk, former head of the Cytochemistry Division of the National Cancer Institute, comments:

> Amygdalin itself contains no ordinarily measurable quantity of prussic acid (syn. hydrocyanic acid, hydrogen cyanide, HCN), and indeed no quantity of acid greater than one part in 10 million when amygdalin is dissolved in neutral water (pH 7), as has been established by many chemists.[1]

The importance of this fact is that, according to the FDA itself, the extracts of almond, peach, and apricot seeds are generally *regarded as safe!*

On August 20, 1975, the FDA issued a "Talk Paper" over the signature of Edward R. Nida. It stated:

> Last spring a cancer patient, now deceased, and her husband sued the government asking that an FDA order prohibiting distribution of Laetrile be vacated. *No such order exists.* [Emphasis added.]

I have in my possession (and have introduced into the court record) a photocopy of a purchase order for Laetrile issued to the Cyto Pharma laboratory in Tijuana, Mexico. It was sent by the prestigious Sloan-Kettering Institute for Cancer Research in New York. Also introduced as evidence is a copy of a cargo

---

[1]"Fact Sheet," *op. cit.*, p. 3.

manifest to Sloan-Kettering from Mr. Sergio del Rio of Tijuana. Both of these Laetrile shipments were passed through U.S. Customs without a hitch.

A great deal of the amygdalin used in this country was imported from Germany by the Spectro Foods Corporation of Montclair, New Jersey. This, too, was cleared through Customs for over a year and a five-per-cent import duty paid on every gram.

On March 28, 1976, the state legislature of Alaska passed a law specifically allowing doctors to use Laetrile in the treatment of cancer, an act that certainly would not have received support if there had been any serious question about Laetrile's legal status at the federal level.

So it is clear that there is no valid federal law against the use of amygdalin or Laetrile. Why, then, does the FDA doggedly pursue its course of harassment?

Part of the answer lies in the nature of the government; or, to be more specific, in the human nature of those individuals who wield governmental power. Nowhere in history has government ever admitted that it was wrong. Government, to survive, must always be right. The moment a government official honestly admits that he has made a serious mistake, he is shown to be incompetent by those who would like to have his job. That's why men in government—even those very high in government—sometimes lie and resort to un-Constitutional acts. It is merely to prevent the world from discovering that they have made a mistake.

In the case of Laetrile, officials at all levels of government have made one of the biggest mistakes of history. I think many of them know it now; and, as the truth spreads to larger numbers of people, their efforts to stop it become both more frantic and unethical. They are fighting, not to protect the public, but to protect themselves.

So that is part of the reason the vast power of government has been set against those of us who dare to use Laetrile, but there is another part that is equally important. I discussed it at some length during my opening remarks to the jury at my fourth trial in the U.S. Circuit Court in San Diego. The date was January 18, 1977. Acting as my own defense attorney, I said:

> Ladies and gentlemen of the jury: You are sitting in judgment of a case that may be one of the most important in American history. The issue is not smuggling, but literally whether medical science is to be frozen by bureaucratic fiat. The lives of millions are in the balance. I am charged with conspiracy to smuggle—but the purpose of this prosecution is not to punish a smuggler but forever to chain the advancement of medical science to political whim. . . .
>
> The logical question now is why everybody would get so excited about a doctor using Vitamin B_{17} in his practice. This is a simple question, but the answer is very complicated. Let me try to make sense out of it for you.
>
> Every year more than 370,000 Americans are killed by cancer. It is by far the most feared of the deadly diseases. Man has, with little success, been looking for a cure to this horrible killer for ages. Much of the research has been sponsored by the American Cancer Society, established long ago by the Rockefeller family and some of its business friends. Since they were in the petroleum and drug businesses they were interested in looking for a solution to the cancer threat that involved the use of synthetic drugs. As it happens, most synthetic drugs have a coal-tar base; that is, they are derivatives of petroleum.
>
> Over the past several decades the American Cancer Society has financed and directed the vast majority of the cancer research in this country through grants. There may or may not have been something sinister in all this, but the point is that if you wanted money to do cancer research you were most likely to get it by looking in an area which involves the use of coal-tar-based chemicals and assorted synthetic medicines.
>
> Maybe they have not been looking in the right place. There is another theory on the prevention and control of cancer. This lies in the

field of orthomolecular medicine. That is a term coined in 1968 by Dr. Linus Pauling, the famous Nobel laureate. The prefix "ortho," from the Greek, means "correct." and "molecular" relates to molecules. According to the Linus Pauling Institute of Science and Medicine, in its *Newsletter*, Volume 1, Number 1:

Orthomolecular medicine is the achievement and preservation of good health and the prevention and treatment of disease by the use of substances that are normally present in the human body; that is, by changing the amounts of those substances in the human body. The vitamins are substances of this sort. One of the goals of orthomolecular medicine is to determine the amounts of various vitamins that are needed to put people in the best of health. Synthetic drugs and other artificial substances are not a part of orthomolecular medicine.

As much as $28 billion is spent each year in the fields of cancer research, detection, and treatment. You could put the portion of this $28 billion which goes into orthomolecular research in your eye and it would not blur your vision. The Bureaucrats, foundation powers, and medical politicians do not intend to be proved wrong. The answer is going to be found in synthetics come hell or high water. In the opinion of those of us in orthomolecular medicine, this means it may never be found at all while Americans continue to die horribly at the rate of 370,000 a year.

Let us take a look at Linus Pauling for a moment. Now, politically, I consider Dr. Pauling to be on the moon, but there is no denying that he is one of the great scientists of this century. And for many years he was the absolute reigning darling of the American scientific establishment. Then about ten years ago, he began looking into diet as a factor in preventing and treating disease. Pauling has set up an institute at Stanford University for the study of orthomolecular medicine. But even Linus Pauling, possibly the most famous living scientist in the world, cannot obtain grants from either the big foundations or the government to carry out his research. Professor Pauling has gone from the penthouse of the scientific establishment to its outhouse. He was forced to buy ads in the *Wall Street Journal* of November 8, 1976, to solicit research funds. The Pauling Institute's solicitation begins:

Our research shows that the incidence and severity of cancer depends upon diet. We urgently want to refine that research, so that it may help to decrease suffering from human cancer.

The U.S. government has absolutely and continually refused to support Dr. Pauling and his colleagues here in this work during the past four years.

I can tell you that if Dr. Pauling were researching in the field of petroleum-based chemicals he would be inundated with funds from both the U.S. Government and the American Cancer Society. But Nobel laureate Linus Pauling, the world's most famous living scientist, has become a pariah. He is now a non-person as far as the U.S. medical establishment is concerned—simply because he believes that a solution to the mystery of cancer lies in the field of diet, and that prevention and treatment can be found through vitamins, minerals, and enzymes. You see, they cannot be patented. Potential profits, therefore, do not justify commercial research.

Probably the most difficult thing to understand about all this is that men of science could be so foolish as to foreclose the avenue suggested by Pauling and others. Cancer is such a horrible disease that it staggers the mind to think that every possibility of finding a means of prevention or remedy is not being exhaustively explored. Cynics have pointed out that with the billions of dollars flowing into cancer research—that is, cancer research of the "right" kind—there is more money to be made looking for a cure than in actually finding it. I believe that the scientists doing actual cancer research hope with all their hearts that they will be successful. Besides the humanitarian aspects involved, whoever finds a cure or preventative for cancer will become one of the most famous people in history. Just as Jonas Salk has become a household word for producing a preventative for polio, the man or woman who beats cancer will become an instant superstar. Wealth and power will lie at his feet.

The trouble is, as I have explained, that scientists are being financed to look for the answer to cancer only within the realm of traditional cancer therapies. They have not been able to get money to investigate the field of nutrition as it relates to cancer—no matter how much we in orthomolecular medicine produce in the way of evidence that they are looking for the needle in the wrong haystack. At the rate things are going, they may never find it. If so, millions of people are going to die agonizing and terrible deaths because of the intransigence springing from politics, bureaucracy, and blind arrogance.

We have no quarrel with those who insist on finding the solution to cancer within the realm of petroleum-based chemicals, although we think they are wrong. What grates us is that these people and their legion of associated bureaucrats and hired propagandists insist that anybody dealing with cancer from any other position is automatically a quack. Now, of course, they do not call Dr. Linus Pauling a quack. They just cut off his funds while shaking their heads and tsk-tsking about what a shame it is that this great man has lost his marbles. But, ladies and gentlemen of the jury, let me remind you that Pauling is dealing in the field of pure research. I have to face the man or woman who is dying of cancer. The doctor is on the front line of this battle, sandwiched in between medical orthodoxy, which would label him a quack, and the patient who is in desperate need. This is why I am in court for the fourth time.

There is an obvious tendency for the federally regulated big drug companies, the medical politicians of the American Cancer Society, and the Food and Drug Administration to act as one big happy family. We all know that many generals and admirals leave the Pentagon and retire to cushy jobs with defense contractors. Then they proceed to negotiate defense contracts with their old chums. This fact of political life has received a fair amount of publicity. What has received virtually no publicity is the fact that the same kind of musical chairs is played among the drug company giants, the American Cancer Society, and the Food and Drug Administration. Much of this, incidentally, has been brought out by Senator William Proxmire of Wisconsin.

What it all means is that, by operating in both the private and public sectors, a powerful clique has a hammerlock on research and treatment in the field of cancer. If you are on their team and play the cancer game their way, you are respectable, and you get public recognition with lots of generous grants. If you are not on their team and persist you will be vilified as a quack preying upon the suffering of others. You will be harassed by every possible branch of government with sensationalists in the mass media treating you like some kind of dope peddler. You can imagine how humiliating and infuriating it is to be faced with such an assault and to know that if you and other medical scientists give in to it you could be signing the death warrants of literally millions.

Not that there are not real quacks in the field of cancer who prey upon ignorance and desperation—black-box charlatans and seedy con men. But it should be clear to even the merest stripling that no legitimate Doctor of Medicine like myself, with a thriving practice and after years of study and faithful service, would give all that up to become a quack and subject himself and his family to the Hell that I am being put through.

I am not trying to imply that everyone connected with the big drug companies, the American Cancer Society, and the FDA is consciously saying to himself: "I don't care how many people die agonizing deaths as long as my career is on the upswing." Nobody is that blatant. But we do know that human beings have an incredible capacity for rationalization of anything which they see as being in their immediate self-interest. If people were not given to rationalization, nobody would smoke. The bars would close down, we would all go on a diet, and the churches would be overflowing. Crime would virtually disappear, and maybe we would all sprout angel wings. But this is not Utopia; it is the real world. People are given to self-deception and self-delusion. Probably even the prosecutor in this case sincerely believes that he is here today to protect the public's interest, justifying on that basis some of the lawyer tricks he has been playing.

My point is that human nature is still human nature, and there is a vast and vested self-interest in the orthodox treatment of cancer that has been endorsed by a massive bureaucracy. These people tend to be unwilling to admit that anyone searching for answers elsewhere can be motivated by any other feelings besides greed and malice. The oil companies want to sell petroleum products to the pharmaceutical companies. The drug companies want to sell their products to doctors and hospitals. Doctors who are trained to do so, and ignorant of other alternatives in indicated cases, want to perform operations and use radiation and chemotherapy. Scientists want grants. Bureaucrats at H.E.W. want to expand their authority by getting the federal government more and more involved in medicine, and they recognize in fear of cancer an excuse for doing so.

All these people have an enormous interest in maintaining the *status quo,* and react with anger and resentment at anyone who challenges their well-financed authority. Collectively, the prejudice and bigotry of their reaction is the defense perimeter of what can only be called the Cancer Establishment. Those of us who dare to differ with this Cancer Establishment become the enemy. That is why I am here in this court today instead of home treating the sick and suffering. . . .

I hope that now you see why I began this introductory statement with the observation that you are acting as the jury in an affair which is far more important than a simple smuggling case. The prosecutor knows I am not a smuggler. He knows he has no case against me. What is going on here is that a physician named John Richardson has challenged the Cancer Establishment.

I have tried to make it clear that the issues involved in the Laetrile controversy are much broader than meet the eye. To the totally uninformed, it is merely a question of faithful public servants attempting to put an end to quackery. To the more careful observer, it appears to be a question of honest disagreement between two opposing points of view. To the real student of the subject, it is but part of the historic battle in which entrenched error and corrupted science attempt to defeat the emergence of a threatening truth. To those with yet a deeper understanding, it is an economic war in which vast cartels utilize captive segments of government to destroy their competition. And to those who can perceive the ultimate truth, it is a struggle between ideologies: collectivism and paternalistic government versus individualism and the right of a free citizen to choose his own destiny.

I rest my case on two invincible arguments. The first is contained in the Constitution of the United States, which I believe is the greatest document of freedom ever penned by man. It still stands, if we will but have faith enough in it to *use* it.

For those who complain that the Constitution is dead or that it means only what the Supreme Court says it means, I offer the second argument. It is the principle of Nuremberg. When Nazi war criminals were accused of genocide, they defended themselves on the basis that they were just following orders and obeying the laws of the Nazi state. The civilized world cried out: "Guilty!" Man is expected to respond to a higher law than that of any state. When the laws of one's government require a man to condemn innocent people to death, he must reject those laws and stand with his conscience. If he does not, then he is no different from the Nazis who were hanged for war crimes.

In the present battle, we do not even have the passion of war to justify our behavior. Yet, in the last few years more people have died needlessly of cancer than all the casualties of all our wars put together.

How much suffering and death are the American people willing to take before they stand up to the bureaucracy? How many physicians must be put into prison before all physicians cry "enough!" to the increasing government control over their profession? How many more Watergates do we need before we realize that mortal men are corrupted by power, and that the solution to one's problems lies not in *increasing* the power of government but in *decreasing* it?

The spirit of resistance is in the air. It is a refreshing breeze, and it gives me great hope. I have resolved to stand alone if need be. But, as I write these final words, I can't help but wonder, is there anyone else out there?

VI

How to Read the Case Histories

by Patricia Griffin, R.N., B.S.

An explanation of the criteria and methodology used in the selection of case histories; general observations regarding the problems and limitations inherent in such a study; and a description of the standard metabolic therapy, including the recommended diet.

Assembling these case histories has been far more difficult than anyone had anticipated. First of all, Dr. Richardson is treating patients, not conducting a research program, and it is virtually impossible to establish a follow-up contact with many former patients. Typically, after their initial course of Laetrile therapy, they improve, go back home, and are never heard from again. Some of them have moved away. Some have gone off their maintenance prescription. Some have returned to orthodox treatments under pressure from their family physician. Some don't want to cooperate in the follow-up study for fear their employers will learn they have cancer and will not promote them. Some are afraid they will become involved with the law for using an "illegal" substance. And many just don't respond to our letter of inquiry because they are too busy. (One lady we couldn't locate, for instance, had been on a cross-country camping trip driving her own recreational vehicle.)

Another hindrance was our insistence on having on file copies of all medical records verifying the existence of cancer in each of the patients discussed. We knew all too well that the skeptics would claim these people never really had cancer in the first place and that we had cured only their hypochondria. Much to our amazement, however, we learned that many patients actually were afraid to write to their family physician for such records—or to have us do so—because they feared that he either would be offended by their seeking treatment elsewhere, or that he would be angry with them for using Laetrile against his specific advice. Some of the best and most dramatic cases were in this category. We did not include them in this book, however, lest they be used by our critics to cast doubt upon the validity of the entire study. The only exceptions to this policy have been a few cases where the patients had previously undergone extensive surgery, radiation, or chemotherapy. Under those conditions it would seem reasonable to accept the patients' word regarding the existence of a firm diagnosis, otherwise it would have constituted gross malpractice for their physicians to subject them to such radical intervention.

Approximately four thousand cancer patients have been treated at the Richardson Clinic. Almost all of them have shown a positive response to their initial course of therapy before returning home. Out of this group, we selected a cross-section of about five hundred for our study. We were able to establish contact and a working relationship with only about two hundred and fifty of these. The cases with the weakest medical histories were discarded, as were those which were overly repetitious. The remainder are contained in this study; but by no means do they represent our entire files. If we had had the benefit of a large, tax-exempt research grant, the means by which our critics often finance their projects, we could have hired a team of interviewers and statisticians to produce an impressive volume with several thousand pages of similar case histories. Until such grants are made available, however, this limited study is the best we can offer.

The use of the names of hospitals in these studies

is exclusively for the purpose of identifying the institution that verified the diagnosis. It is *not* intended to imply that these institutions are favorably inclined toward Laetrile.

It is not customary in medical journals or books to use patients' names. The only ones who will be identified in this book are those who have consented to have their photographs, X-rays, or other medical records published in this volume.

In passing, it should be noted that the attitude of many physicians whose patients ultimately came to the Richardson Clinic has not been one of cooperation. Some doctors have been openly hostile, and a few even have resorted to letters of extreme personal vilification. It is partly for this reason that we have not used the names of specific doctors in this study. The other reason is that many of these case histories involve patients who have suffered more from their original therapy than they did from the cancer. In other words, the facts presented here do not always reflect favorably upon the original physicians, and to use their names would serve no constructive purpose. All names and documents are on file, however, and will be furnished to anyone who has a legitimate reason to know.

Admittedly, one of the weaknesses of this study is the shortage of cases involving five-year survival or longer. The obvious reason is that Dr. Richardson began using Laetrile only in 1971, and, at first, the number of cancer patients under his care was very small. It was not until about 1973 that the clinic began to handle a large patient load. Consequently, most of these case histories fall into the one-and-a-half to three-year category, with only a few at the five-year level. It should be noted, however, that the literature of orthodox medicine is loaded with studies involving only one or one-and-a-half-year survivals. While these shorter periods are not so conclusive, they *are* significant—especially in large numbers—and should not be ignored. Furthermore, if there is sufficient response to warrant the effort, we plan to update and expand this study based on continuing experience.

It is possible that not all the patients whose histories are presented in this book will be alive five or ten years from now. Some will pass away of heart attack, some in accidents, some from the delayed effects of radiation or toxic chemotherapy, and some, of course, from the damage already caused by their cancer before starting the Laetrile therapy. But bear in mind that the majority of these cases were classified as "terminal" before they ever came to the Richardson Clinic. That some of them will not make it is to be expected. That *any* of them should be alive a year or two later is a major victory for Laetrile. That virtually all of them should experience a loss of pain, a return of strength, and a dramatic improvement in the quality of life—for as long as that life may be theirs—is an enviable achievement that consensus medicine so far has failed to match.

I think it is important to record here also that, out of approximately two hundred and fifty personal letters received from patients and former patients in the course of preparing these case histories, only two have complained of their care; and one of these still spoke favorably of Laetrile. This is a dissatisfaction ratio of less than one per cent, and I rather doubt if there are many cancer specialists among Dr. Richardson's critics who would care to try to match that record.

Some medical professionals may criticize the case histories as containing too much anecdotal material relating to the psychosocial impact of the cancer diagnosis and subsequent treatment. Patients' problems, however, do not cease when the lump or bump has been removed—far from it.

The fact that individuals sometimes are fired from their jobs as soon as it becomes known they have cancer may weigh as heavily on these patients as the consequences of surgery, radiation, and chemotherapy.

When a man has his testes removed at the suggestion of his doctor to "control" his cancer, he has more problems than simple wound healing. If a woman's husband can no longer respond romantically to her because of his reaction to the absence of one or both of her breasts, then the quality of those lives has been changed drastically and the hope of life extension has been purchased at a terrible price.

Orthodox therapy, (surgery, radiation, and chemotherapy) because of its lump or bump concept of cancer, is required to view the elimination of that lump or bump as the only meaningful measure of its success. Psychosocial factors are not prime considerations. The sincere, concerned, and dedicated physician could not live with himself if he were to think too much about the problems he creates when, for instance, he must remove someone's nose. We feel we must bring these problems into focus—in addition to presenting medical data—if the value of metabolic therapy, as an alternative to present modalities, is to be fully realized.

I must admit to entering this project with my own bias. I knew that Laetrile was of value. I was inclined, however, toward the "magic bullet" theory that Laetrile and Laetrile alone was the answer. I underestimated the need for pancreas enzymes, additional vitamins and minerals, and the vegetarian diet. I understood the rationale, but I did not fully appreciate its importance.

Because of my previous convictions regarding the value of animal protein, I suppose, subconsciously, I wanted to find this "faddish" diet as unnecessary adjunct to a successful metabolic regimen. The case histories were powerful persuaders to the contrary. It appears that the cancer patient is no more likely to respond to Laetrile alone than is the severe diabetic likely to be symptom-free by taking insulin and then consuming banana splits, whipped-cream pie, and sweet soft drinks. I had to conclude that, for the so-called terminal patient, adherence to the diet is literally a life or death requirement.

It is my opinion, based on personal interviews and on correspondence with Richardson Clinic patients, that the reason the men with cancer of the prostate—even those with evidence of metastasis to lymph nodes or bone—do so very well, as a group, is that they are the most consistently faithful to all aspects of the regimen, including the diet.

It seems to me that, if the drive to maintain a state of general health were as strong in *all* patients, male or female, as the drive to preserve potency appears to be in patients with cancer of the prostate, there would be an increase in survival rates that would amaze not only the skeptic but the Laetrile enthusiast as well.

The details of each patient's treatment at the Richardson Clinic have not been spelled out because, *in general,* metabolic therapy is fairly standardized. (The rationale for the diet and vitamin regimen is described in Chapter One.) Rather than repeat the listing of each vitamin, mineral, and other supplement as a part of every case history, they will be summarized below:

1. THE DIET—principally fresh fruits, vegetables, seeds, nuts, and grains. All animal protein, including dairy products, is excluded.
2. TOBACCO, ALCOHOL, and COFFEE are not to be used.
3. LAETRILE (Vitamin B_{17}) INJECTIONS—

SCHEDULE	INJECTIONS	AMOUNT	FREQUENCY
First Month	I.V.	6-9 gms. or more	1 per day for 20 days
Second Month	I.V. or I.M.	3 gms.	3 per week for 4 weeks
Third Month	I.V. or I.M.	3 gms.	2 per week for 4 weeks
Fourth to Eighteenth Month	I.V. or I.M.	3 gms.	1 per week for 1 to 1½ years or longer

4. LAETRILE (Vitamin B_{17}) TABLETS—one to four 500 mg. tablets are taken on the days the patient is *not* receiving an injection of Laetrile. Two tablets per day is the usual dosage during the first year. Most patients will continue taking tablets for the rest of

their lives. Some will use 100 mg. tablets and supplement with apricot kernels. *The kernels must be taken at a different time during the day than the Laetrile tablets.*

5. PANCREATIC ENZYME TABLETS—two to four tablets, four times daily.
6. VITAMIN B_{15} (PANGAMIC ACID)—50 mg. three times daily.
7. VITAMIN C—750 mg. to 2,000 mg. daily.
8. AMINO ACID TABLETS (Ag/Pro)—three to nine tablets daily to compensate for reduced intake of animal protein.
9. CHELATED MINERALS—dosage dependent upon the type and extent of deficiency revealed by hair analysis.
10. THERAPEUTIC VITAMINS AND MINERALS (Supergran)—one or two capsules daily.
11. VITAMIN E—800 I.U. to 1,200 I.U. daily.
12. LIQUID PROTEIN—two to four tablespoons daily. This protein is in a "predigested" form providing basic amino acids that do not require the action of pancreas enzymes for their use by the body. (This is used by those patients who are not taking Ag/Pro tablets.)
13. ADDITIONAL VITAMINS AND MINERALS—to be recommended where necessary in special cases.

The Richardson Clinic's metabolic regimen is by its very nature humane. It reflects the philosophy of Hippocrates, the Father of Medicine, who taught his students, "First do no harm."

VII

The Case Histories

by Patricia Griffin, R.N., B.S.

The Richardson Cancer Clinic Experience

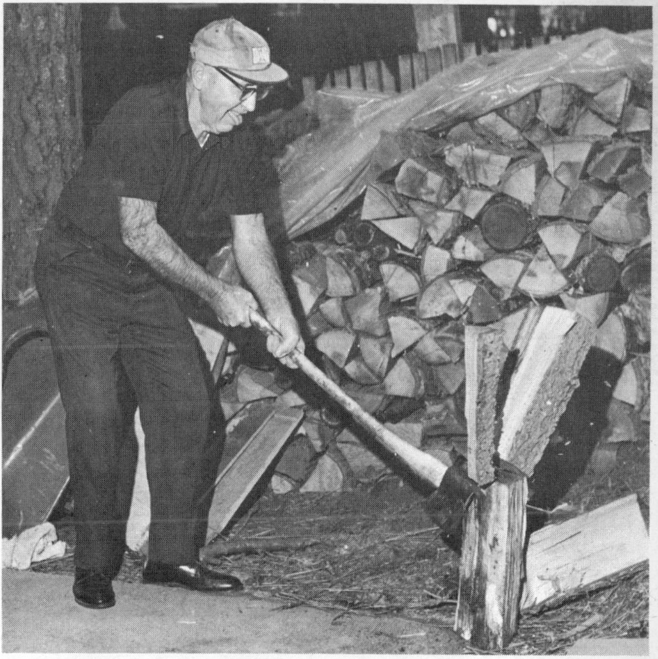

Photo by Jack Lauck

John Peterson (case 107) had been given less than a year to live as a result of inoperable cancer of the prostate. His disease progressed rapidly, causing intense and constant pain. His body jerked in spasms, he began bleeding from the rectum, and often passed out from pain and weakness. It was at this point that he turned to Laetrile.

Within 30 days of his first injection he was able to drive his own car and lead a near-normal life. He is shown here two years later, enjoying one of his favorite activities.

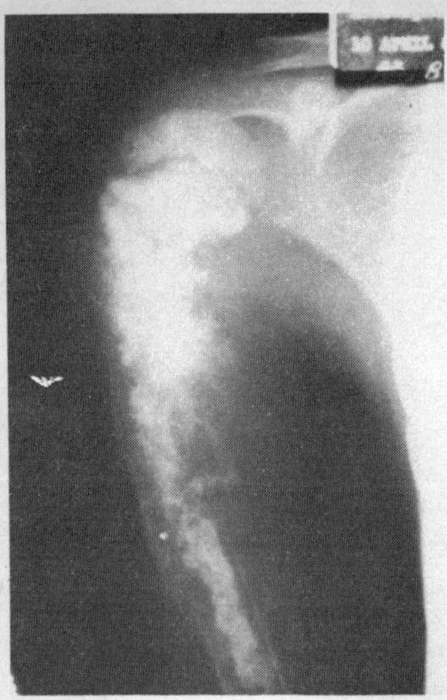

Shane Horton (case 150) was six years old when he developed osteosarcoma of the right upper arm and of the spine. This was confirmed both by X-ray and bone-marrow biopsy. His doctors advised that there was no hope. It was at this point that his parents elected Laetrile therapy.

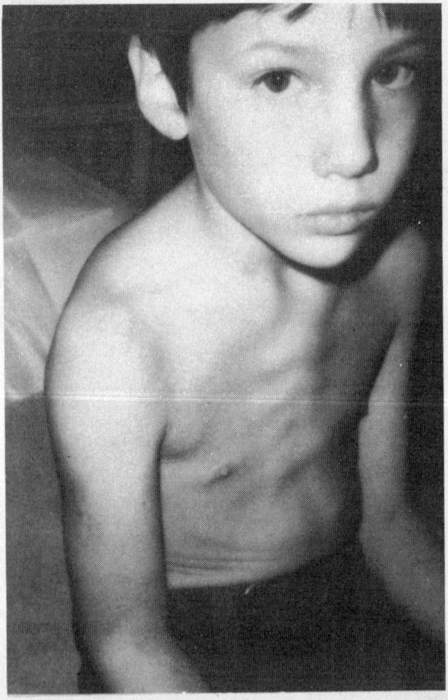

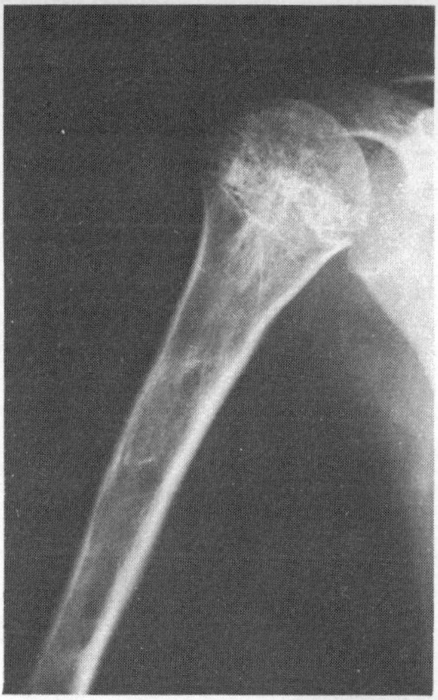

Three years after beginning Laetrile therapy, all evidence of bone cancer had vanished, and Shane was enjoying the life of a completely normal nine-year-old.

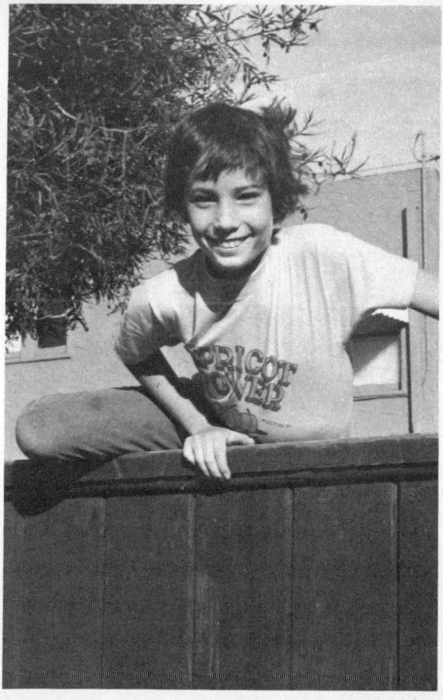

Photo by Steve Richardson

Dr. John Richardson is met at the San Francisco airport by the press corps. A doctor becomes newsworthy when he abandons orthodox therapies and challenges the cancer establishment.

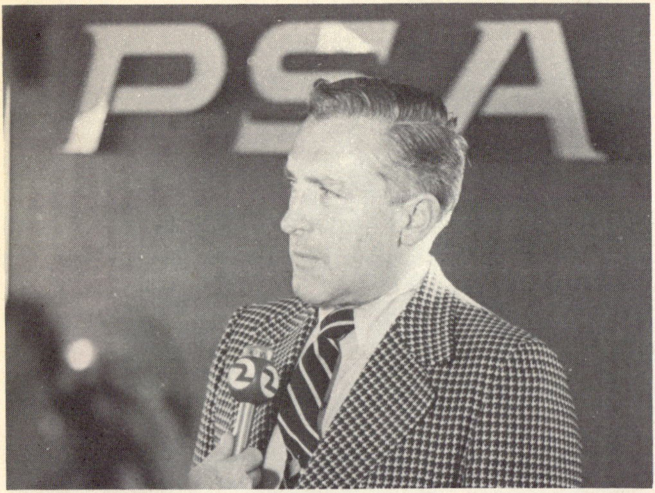

Photo by Steve Richardson

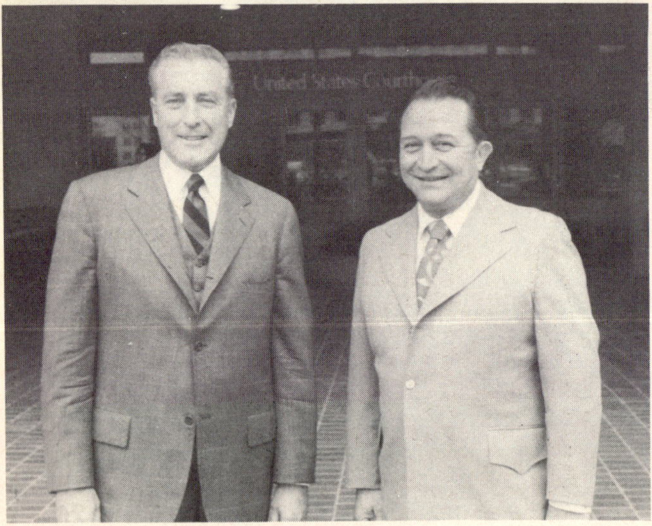

Photo by G. Edward Griffin

Dr. Richardson and Ralph Bowman, his office manager and long-time friend, pause confidently in front of the Federal Courthouse in San Diego, where they are challenging the government's restrictions on the use of Laetrile.

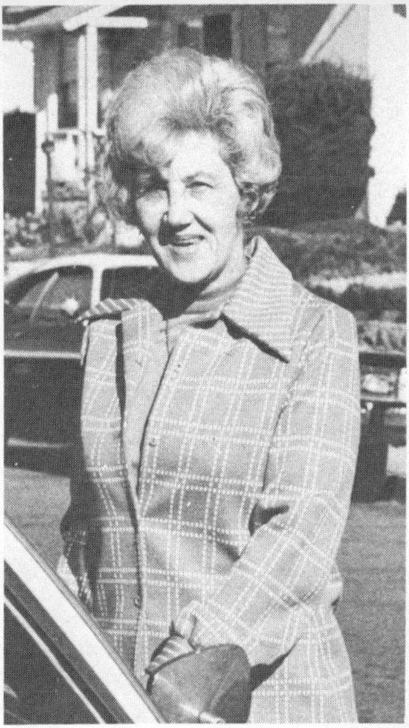

Photo by Steve Richardson

Mrs. Lorette Lau, left (case 152), was told by her doctor in 1975 that, unless she submitted to radiation or chemotherapy as treatment for her cancer of the ovary, she could not live longer than a year. She declined his advice and came to the Richardson Clinic for metabolic therapy instead. She has responded beautifully and continues to enjoy good health.

Mrs. Lorraine Ford, right (case 115), suffered from inoperable cancer of the liver, with previous cancer of the breast. Statistically, most patients in this category are dead within six months of diagnosis. After the failure of chemotherapy, she turned to Laetrile as a last resort in December of 1974. Today she leads an active and normal life.

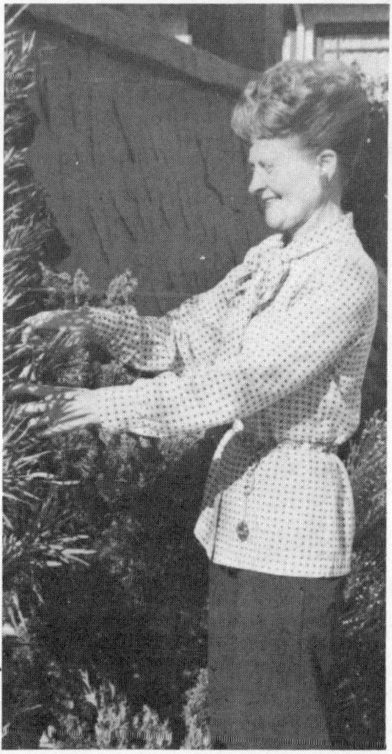

Photo by Steve Richardson

Ben Reynolds (case 106) is enjoying good health with his wife four and one-half years after he was diagnosed as having chronic lymphatic leukemia. Except for three days on chemotherapy, he has had no treatment other than metabolic therapy including Laetrile.

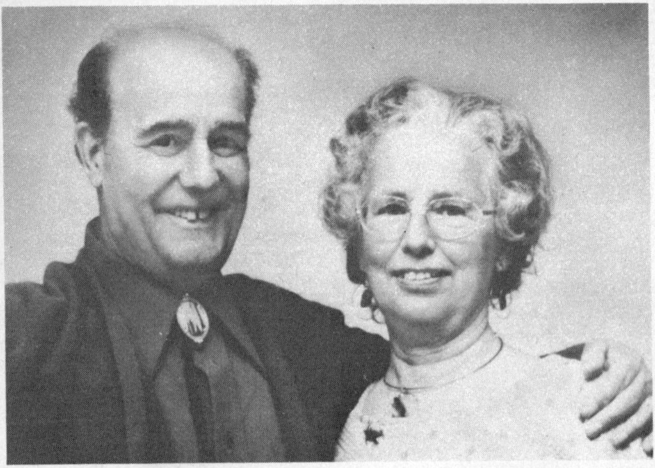

Photo by Steve Richardson

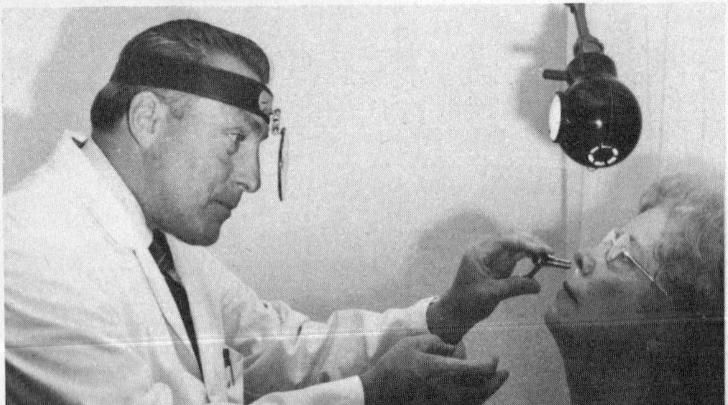

Photo by Steve Richardson

Dr. John Richardson is not a "lump or bump" doctor. He views the malignant tumor merely as a symptom of the disease called cancer, not the disease itself. As long as orthodox medicine continues to treat only the symptom, it can never hope to conquer the cause.

Mrs. Linda Barton, below (case 133), developed cancer of the cervix, confirmed by biopsy, in 1975. Rejecting surgery, she chose, instead, metabolic therapy, including Laetrile. Subsequent tests have shown no trace of cancer.

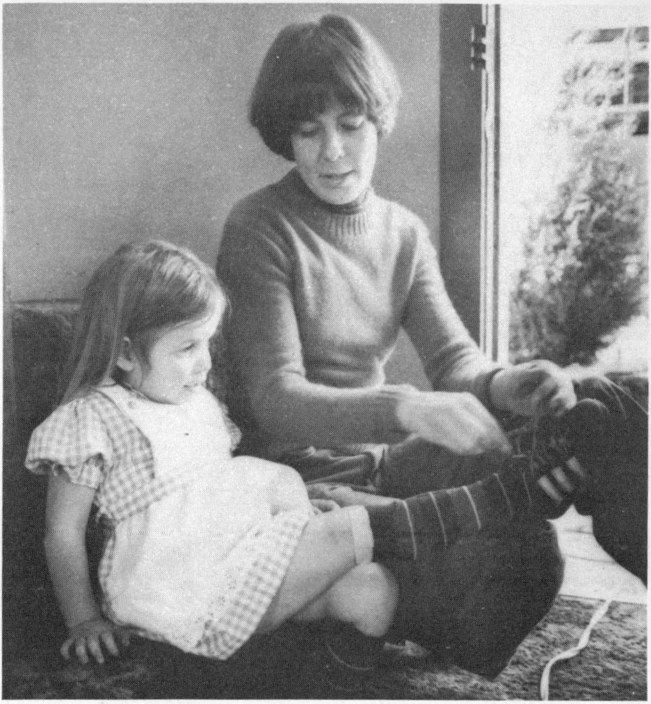

Photo by Steve Richardson

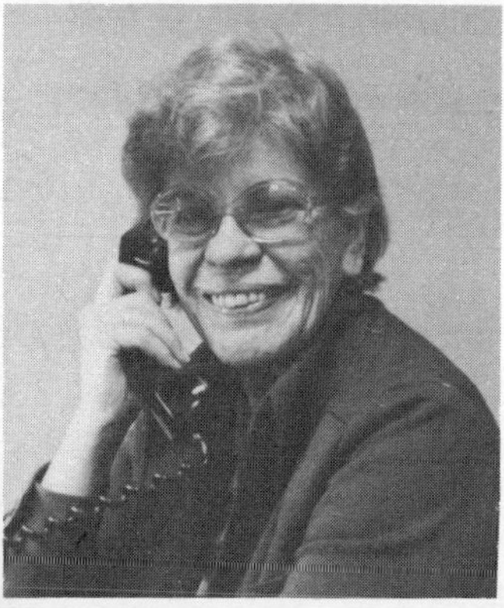

Mrs. Thelma Mosca, left (case 122), was diagnosed as having cancer of the cervix in January of 1975 and was slated for surgery including a radical hysterectomy. She changed her mind about the surgery and decided to try Laetrile instead. At this point her doctor told her she would be dead within three months. Two years after beginning Laetrile therapy she is leading an active and rewarding life of involvement in community service.

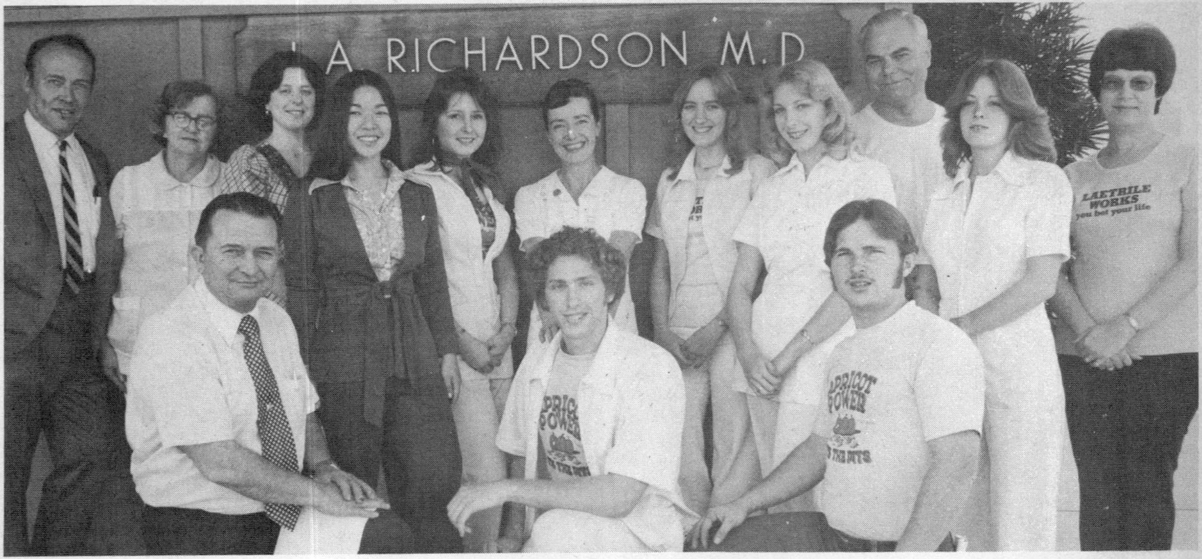

The Richardson Clinic staff as of January, 1977: (standing, L to R) William Brodie, M.D., Mary Botelho, Joanna Ketner, Joie Toyotome, Gail Bowman, Angela Gillmer, R.N., Trudy Prince, Becky Richardson, Bela Veress, Jannell Garrett, Janice Eby; (kneeling, L to R) Ralph Bowman, Steve Richardson, Matt Bowman; (not shown) Elmer Thomassen, M.D., Laura Bowman, John Richardson, M.D.

CANCER OF THE BREAST

Two out of every three patients with cancer of the breast who do not use Laetrile *but choose instead to submit to orthodox therapies will be dead within five years.*[1] *If a cancerous lump is present for one month only, fifty per cent of patients will have metastasis.*[2] *The following Laetrile case histories should be read with this in mind.*

M110MX: Cancer of the Breast

In July, 1974, this fifty-year-old woman sought medical attention because of a lump in her left breast. Subsequent mammogram and needle biopsy were both negative. The mammogram report concluded, however:

> Clinically palpable firm mass in the lower portion of the left breast which radiographically presents as an ill defined increase in density not to unlike that of fibrocystic change. The clinical feel of the lesion, however, warrants biopsy.

The patient decided to have the lump removed but would not sign a surgery consent for removal of the breast in the event the lesion was cancer.

Pathology report stated in part:

---

[1]*Clinical Oncology for Medical Students and Physicians, op. cit.,* p. 99.
[2]*Ibid.* p. 91.

Microscopic: . . . In some areas the tumor occurs as nests of cells which extend into the surrounding adipose tissue. The tumor extends to the margins of resection.
Microscopic Diagnosis:
Infiltrating Ductal Carcinoma, Left Breast.

The fact that the tumor extended "to the margins of resection" tells us that not all of it was removed. Because of this, the doctors urged her to have her left breast amputated. The probable need for cobalt therapy following surgery also was suggested.

This woman decided that she preferred to try metabolic therapy including Laetrile. Treatment was begun in August, 1974. She began the standard twenty-day course of therapy, receiving 6 to 9 grams of Laetrile I.V. per day. This was supplemented by a regimen of pancreatic enzymes and a broad spectrum of vitamins and minerals. She began the recommended animal-protein-free diet and has remained on it since that time. She has rejected all forms of orthodox therapy.

To the surprise of her original physician, this patient's cancer has not reappeared, even though it is certain that malignant tissue remained after her excisional biopsy. She continues to lead an entirely normal life with no evidence of cancer.

F161W: Cancer of the Left Breast with Metastases to the Lymph Nodes

This woman was fifty-three years old at the time she was admitted to the hospital for evaluation of changes in her left breast. The date was February 6, 1975.

On her hospital admission history, she stated she had noted about December 12, 1974, that the nipple of her left breast was pulled back from its normal position. On examination, the doctor admitting her to the hospital felt the lymph nodes and stated that there was an "indefinite mass."

The patient had surgery the following day. The area beneath the left breast was biopsied, and the pathologist reported "infiltrating ductal cell carcinoma." The doctor then proceeded to do a radical amputation of the left breast. The pathology report dated February 10, 1975, stated in part:

> *Gross:*
> Numerous enlarged, obviously involved lymph nodes are present.
> *Microscopic:*
> There are ten slides and multiple sections. . . . Examination reveals the presence of metastases in 8 of 13 examined lymph nodes. Metastases are noted in the two highest nodes.
> *Pathologic Diagnosis:*
> Left breast, infiltrating duct cell carcinoma in large part scirrhous type with metastases to 8 of 13 examined lymph nodes.

The fact that cancer had spread to the highest lymph nodes examined is generally considered a bad sign in terms of patient survival.

The patient states she saw her doctor again on March 24, 1975. Apparently he felt her prognosis was so grave that he didn't even bother recommending radiation or chemotherapy. He indicated there was little hope for recovery and said simply, "You'll just have to face it." In a letter to the Richardson Clinic, the patient described her reaction to the interview with her local doctor:

> I was appalled. There was nothing more to be done, no recommendations, and most of all, no one with whom I could ask questions or discuss the situation.
>
> I recalled seeing a film about Laetrile. My husband called the person who had shown the film here in Grass Valley, California, and after discussing it with her and after reading several books on the subject, we decided that vitamin therapy was the answer.

The patient came to the Richardson Clinic on March 24, 1975. She received 9 gms. of Laetrile I.V. every day for twenty days, and then the dosage was gradually reduced. Mineral intake was balanced based on her hair analysis. Blood studies were essentially normal. Bio-assays were: (1) 3-24-75, 26.7; (2) 6-18-75, 18.7; (3) 10-2-75, 15.1; (4) 1-12-76, 14.5; (5) 3-29-76, 15.0; (6) 8-10-76, 21.4.[1]

Currently the patient is taking two 500 mg. tablets of Laetrile per day and one 3 gm. I.V. injection of Laetrile per month. She is maintaining her vegetarian diet with the exception of occasional servings of fish or chicken.

It has been more than two years since this patient was abandoned by orthodox medicine. Under metabolic therapy she continues in excellent health. She does all of her housework, helps in the yard, looks after her family and cares for her elderly mother, who lives nearby.

K132MH: Cancer of the Breast with Seeding

This woman went to a clinic in Great Falls, Montana, for a physical examination in May, 1974. Examination revealed what appeared to be cancer. Mrs. K. had a left modified radical mastectomy for "infiltrating ductal carcinoma" (cancer). Two of the eleven lymph nodes were involved with metastatic tumor.

Following the mastectomy, the patient received 4500 rads of cobalt therapy to the left paraclavicular region and the internal mammary areas (collar bone and breast bone areas) in fifteen divided doses over a period of three weeks. She was seen by her doctor at regular intervals during 1975.

She noted some bumps developing in the area of her previous surgery and radiation and returned to her doctor in January, 1976.

In a letter to the Richardson Clinic dated April 7, 1976, the doctor stated in part:

---

[1]See appendix for normals.

> I examined them [the growths] and there were about 2-3 definite nodules in the area of the previous mastectomy. I biopsied some of the nodules and this showed metastatic adenocarcinoma consistent with infiltrating ductular malignancy [cancer].

The patient states the doctor told her she could not have any more radiation and that he did not plan to put her on chemotherapy. It was decided to put her on a course of hormone therapy, instead. She was informed, however, that such therapy was not a cure and, in view of her cancer's return to the old site, there was little orthodox medicine could do for her.

The patient stated in a letter to the Richardson Clinic, March 26, 1976:

> I took them [the pills] a little, but they were Stilbesterol, and I knew the FDA had ordered the cattle feeders not to use it as implants in cattle, because the meat from cattle which had been on the hormone might cause cancer in humans.

The patient continued on Stilbesterol for only a few weeks more and then concluded she should stop taking what she saw as a cancer-causing substance. She stated that the Stilbesterol caused her abdomen to swell, that she was unable to control her urine, and that, although past her menopause, she began to menstruate again.

The patient came to the Richardson Clinic and began metabolic therapy February 3, 1976. Only a little over one year has passed since the return of cancer to the original site of surgery and radiation. It is too early, therefore, to come to definite conclusions regarding the efficacy of metabolic therapy in her case. It should be noted, however, that most patients under such circumstances experience a rapid decline and, at the end of one year, either are deceased or are facing a severe confrontation with their disease. By contrast, this patient's disease appears to be completely controlled and she is enjoying a normal life.

B157M: Cancer of Both Breasts

This woman was fifty years old at the time of her first radical mastectomy in June, 1967. The patient states the doctor assured her they "got it all."

A second radical mastectomy was performed in the same Michigan hospital in 1974. The patient was told at the time of her second breast amputation that it would be necessary for her to have cobalt therapy, and when the cobalt treatments were completed she would have to have her uterus and ovaries removed.

She left her home in Michigan at her doctor's suggestion and went to a Buffalo, N.Y., hospital to prepare for subsequent treatments. The patient had this to say about her treatment in New York:

> I went to Buffalo believing I would receive excellent care because it was reputed to have a good reputation. . . . From the moment I entered the door I felt like a number. I was never taken into an office for a consultation with a doctor about my case. I was sent to a nuclear clinic and told to disrobe and sit on a table. The two doctors who came in did not speak to me, only to each other. The exams without explanation or consultation continued for two weeks. . . .

Later, after conferring with two other doctors in the same hospital who were not associated with the nuclear medicine department, Mrs. B. concluded she did not want cobalt. According to the patient, there were numerous phone calls to her home from various physicians urging her to come back and begin treatment. It was made clear to her that, if she did not submit to radiation, her chances of survival were almost zero. The patient stated, "My feeling about this entire experience was that I was being clawed back into a cage at the nuclear clinic." She returned to Michigan frustrated and disillusioned.

By June, 1975, three small lumps had appeared on the site of the scar of the biopsy which had preceded the second radical mastectomy.

The lumps which had appeared in June, 1975,

and one lymph node were finally removed in December, 1975, at Hermann Hospital, Houston, Texas. The pathology diagnosis stated:

1. Skin with metastatic well differentiated adenocarcinoma extending into subcutaneous tissue.
2. Lymph node with metastatic well differentiated adenocarcinoma.

According to the patient, the physician who performed the surgery in December, 1975, advised the patient's husband that if it were his own wife he would insist on cobalt therapy.

The patient for a second time decided against cobalt.

About this time she had heard of Laetrile and concluded she would try nutritional therapy instead. She began treatments on February 4, 1976. Within just a few days, she noticed a general improvement in her stamina and sense of well-being. Her return to apparent good health since that time has been impressive, especially in view of the fact that she has not always adhered strictly to the prescribed levels of Laetrile or to the recommended diet.

Psychological scars, however, remain. In a recent letter to the Richardson Clinic, the patient stated:

> My only pain has been the result of mutilating and unnecessary surgery. The vegetarian diet distresses me because, at this point in one's life, there are few pleasures remaining to us *and being disfigured makes a dismal difference in any other source of joy.*

In spite of the sad consequences of previous orthodox therapy, the patient has expressed gratitude not only to be alive and well but also to have escaped the probable pain and further disfigurement of radiation.

I125M: Cancer of the Breast

This patient was admitted to General Rose Hospital in Denver, Colorado, for a right radical mastectomy, which was performed on October 30, 1974. She was hospitalized for six weeks following surgery because of an infection at the operative site.

Following surgery, she received radiation from November 27, 1974, to February 20, 1975. During that time, the treatments had to be discontinued for a period of ten days because of body burns.

Upon completion of radiation therapy, the patient was scheduled to start chemotherapy. She had only two shots and discontinued the treatment.

In a letter written by the patient to the Richardson Clinic she describes her local doctor's response to the idea of Laetrile:

> Dr. [name omitted] did the mastectomy and planned the radiation and chemotherapy. However, after two injections of chemotherapy, I walked off the entire mess except to complete paying the bills. . . .
>
> I had read about Laetrile and wanted to discuss this with my doctor. He threw the book, turned red, and yelled, "This is no damn good." . . .
>
> March 10, 1975, I began vitamin therapy. For the first time, I began to feel normal and enjoy being human once again. I have continued the Laetrile shots, the vitamins, and the cancer diet faithfully since March 10, 1975, and it is now March 4, 1976. I do all my normal work, sleep eight hours each night, have much energy, and enjoy life and friends once again.
>
> I have confidence in my vitamin therapy. The surgery and radiation made me feel like a stumbling zombie. I feel like a healthy individual since vitamin therapy.

B145C: Cancer of the Breast

In August, 1974, this thirty-four-year-old woman began to have pain in her left arm, for which her family doctor was unable to find a cause. The patient discovered a lump on her left breast in March, 1975. She states that she returned to her family doctor, who advised her there was no lump; rather, she was feeling the side of her breast.

Three months later, however, the patient sought the advice of her gynecologist, who said there *was* a lump on her breast and advised her to see a surgeon. Following several consultations, the patient was admitted to the hospital, where a radical left breast removal was performed on August 11, 1975.

The surgery report states in part: "On dissecting the tissue away from the highest axillary structures on the chest wall above and behind the axillary structures, tumor and metastases were noted." The report stated that all of the main tumor was removed, but no mention was made of the metastases.

The pathology report from St. Joseph's Hospital in Denver, Colorado, states the final diagnosis as: "Infiltrating ductal carcinoma. Left radical mastectomy with residual intraductal carcinoma [cancer not removed by surgery] and axillary lymph node metastases."

The patient's husband was advised that the cancer had invaded the shoulder area and that the surgeons were unable to cut out all the cancer. Radiation and chemotherapy were both advised, and the probability of subsequent need to remove the patient's ovaries was also discussed.

The patient and her husband decided that she should come to the Richardson Clinic for metabolic therapy instead.

Metabolic therapy including Laetrile was begun September 10, 1975. In a letter dated March 30, 1976, the patient summarizes her experience in part as follows:

> After about the third or fourth shot, the pain in my arm, which had not gone away even after surgery, was gone, and I could use my arm in a fairly normal way. I felt that any kind of therapy which was constructive had to do more good than destructive therapy.

Although this patient is known to have had extensive mestastases at the inception of metabolic therapy, and, thus, her prognosis (under orthodox therapy) would have been extremely unfavorable, she has responded beautifully. Her general health and vitality have improved, and her disease appears to be satisfactorily controlled, inasmuch as she remains symptom-free more than one and one-half years after the incomplete removal of her cancer.

CANCER OF THE LUNG

Eight out of every ten patients with cancer of the Lung who do not use Laetrile *but choose instead to submit to orthodox therapy, will be dead within one year. Ninety-five out of every one hundred patients with cancer of the lung will be dead five years following diagnosis—if they choose only orthodox therapy.*[1] *The following Laetrile case histories should be viewed against this background.*

L118L: Metastatic Cancer of the Left Lung and Pleura and Probable Cancer of the Liver

This woman was sixty-five years old when her symptoms first appeared in July, 1975. She had left shoulder pain and pain on the left side of her chest. Chest X-rays were normal. Alkaline phosphatase was slightly elevated.

In August, 1975, she returned to her doctor again because of increased left-sided chest pain and pain in her left breast. Chest X-ray was normal. Dorsal spine X-ray taken in left lateral position showed pleural fluid. This confirmed the diagnosis of left subpulmonic effusion (the escape of fluid into an area below the lung).

On September 15, 1975, the patient was hospitalized because of almost constant left-sided chest pain. Admission also showed a nodule on her thyroid. Blood

---

[1]*Clinical Oncology for Medical Students and Physicians, op. cit.*, p. 99.

test revealed a change from same tests six weeks earlier. Significant findings were: hemoglobin 11.2, hematocrit 33, SGOT 100 (lab high normal, 35), alkaline phosphatase 160 (lab high normal, 85), G.G.T.P. 228 (lab high normal, 18). Her liver was not enlarged.

On September 19, 1975, the subpulmonic pleural effusion was tapped and fluid removed. The fluid contained protein 4.5 gms/liter, serum albumin 4 gms/liter. Cytology on the fluid was reported as being "consistent with well-differentiated papillary adenocarcinoma [cancer]."

The impression at time of hospital admission (September 15, 1975) was "Metastatic adenocarcinoma involving the left pleura and liver from unknown primary."

The nodule on the thyroid was removed and found *not* to be cancerous. The patient was discharged three weeks later on October 4, 1975.

The patient was hospitalized again from November 3, 1975, through November 7, 1975.

Admission history states in part:

> It was decided [during the previous admission] the likely primary site was either the pancreas, or perhaps bowel or lung and it was elected to treat her with weekly injections of 5-FU. After four treatments there was noted some chest discomfort, and X-rays taken about 10 days ago . . . showed a significant increase in left pleural effusion with small loculated areas of peripneumothorax . . . She is easily fatigued, and has had shortness of breath, and has noticed an increase in abdominal girth. Because of the treatment failure and an attempt again to locate the primary, she is being admitted for pleural biopsy and instillation of nitrogen mustard into the pleural cavity.

On admission the patient's liver was palpable on deep inspiration two finger breadths below the right costal margin.

Pathology report of the pleural biopsy was negative. On November 3, 1975, however, despite the negative biopsy, 11mg. of nitrogen mustard was instilled into the pleural space because of the previous finding of cancer cells in the pleural fluid. Liver biopsy was negative, but the patient was presumed to have cancer of the liver based on the blood study findings.

Discharge diagnosis was, "Cancer of the lung involving the left pleura and possibly the liver, probable metastatic adenocarcinoma, possibly mesothelioma."

This doctor considered her to have inoperable cancer of the lung and probably cancer of the liver.

She states she received weekly infusion of 5-FU, 800 mg. IV at approximately ten-day intervals from November 14, 1975, through January 14, 1976. The patient stated, "My doctor said that I had about a year to live. Knowing that chemotherapy was not a cure, I decided to try Laetrile, feeling hopeful that it would help."

The patient stopped taking 5-FU on January 14, 1976, and began a program of metabolic therapy including Laetrile on February 3, 1976.

Cancer of the lung patients have an over-all survival time of six to nine months. This includes those who can have their tumor "successfully" removed. Chemotherapy is not considered to cure cancer, only to palliate it. Nitrogen mustard has been shown to increase the median survival of patients with lung cancer *at best* by only two and one-half months.[1] Non-operable cancer of the liver patients are usually dead in six months.[2]

The patient was readmitted to the hospital in March, 1976, one month after beginning metabolic therapy. Her complaint was severe pain in the abdomen. The diagnosis was compacted bowels. The patient states, "At that time there was found no enlargement of

---

[1]Green, Humphrey, Chase and Patno. "Alkylating Agents in Bronchogenic Carcinoma", *American Journal of Medicine* 46:516, 1969.
[2]Schwartz, *Surgical Disease of the Liver* (McGraw Hill, New York, 1964). Also, *Clinical Oncology op. cit.*, p. 148.

the tumor and no fluid. Doctor wasn't very pleased with me taking vitamin therapy but was pleased with my condition."

This is a common reaction, particularly among family doctors who may have known and cared for the patient a number of years. They cannot give vitamin therapy any credit because *their* teachers keep insisting it doesn't work. So they respond that they do not approve of what the patient is doing, but they are pleased with the progress.

This patient's symptoms began in July, 1975. Diagnosis was made in September, 1975. Chemotherapy was terminated in January, 1976. Metabolic therapy was begun February, 1976. The patient has responded beautifully and continues with no pain, and in good health. If she were the "average" lung cancer patient, she would have been dead well before the end of 1976. Only twenty per cent of lung cancer patients survive a year, and that, supposedly, is the group on whom surgical removal of the tumor was successful. We were unable to locate survival figures for the patients with more serious inoperable lung cancer, as was the case with this patient, but, presumably, the statistics would be even more unfavorable.

M136TB: Cancer of Both Lungs, Previous Cancer of the Bone

This young man was seventeen years old when his symptoms first began. In December of 1973, he complained of pain in his left knee. X-rays revealed what was first thought to be a torn ligament; later a second doctor decided that the lesion looked like it might be a tumor. The patient states, "When my parents told me the news, my first thought was 'cancer,' and that I was going to lose my leg."

The patient was admitted to Union Hospital in Terre Haute, Indiana. Preparations were made to perform a biopsy. According to the patient, an hour before the planned surgery, the surgeon recommended that the patient go instead to Mayo Clinic because there it would be possible to receive immediate confirmation as to whether the tumor was cancer.

The patient proceeded to Mayo Clinic, and on January 16, 1974, the diagnosis of bone cancer being established, the left leg was amputated above the knee. The patient tolerated the surgery well but was advised to have chest X-rays every three months following surgery because of the possibility of cancer reappearing in the lungs.

The reports were negative until May, 1975, at which time two spots were noted in one lung and one spot in the other.

Surgery was performed at Mayo Clinic in May, 1975, and two cancerous tumors were removed from each lung.

The patient was placed on chemotherapy for five months. He describes his feelings about what he went through in this way:

> I lost all of my hair. While taking the therapy I had to stay in St. Marys Hospital for three days at a time. During those three days, I couldn't eat a thing and was sick to my stomach constantly. It was pure "hell," and knowing now what I know about the treatment, I wouldn't encourage anyone to go through it. I would be more proud to die [at seventeen].

While the patient was on chemotherapy, another spot, suspicious of malignancy, showed up on chest X-rays.

It was at this point that the young man and his parents decided to look into Laetrile as an alternative.

The family left Indiana and came to California to the Richardson Clinic for a three-week stay in December, 1975. The young man describes his reaction to the initial course of therapy in these words:

> Although I didn't feel any physical change right away, my mind was more at ease than it had been for some time. I was treated like I was just

> as normal as anyone walking on this earth—what I mean is, they didn't treat me like I was deathly sick, but they treated me like I was going to get well.
>
> I feel very lucky to have parents who were able to take me all the way to California.

Since 1975 the patient has adhered to the metabolic regimen, including Laetrile and other vitamins, an animal-protein-free diet, and pancreatic enzymes. Under orthodox therapy, his statistical chance for surviving even one year would have been close to zero. Yet, now, well over a year since he began metabolic therapy, it appears that his disease is controlled satisfactorily. In a letter to us only six months following commencement of his metabolic therapy, the patient wrote:

> Before my leg was amputated, I did lots of skiing, hunting, and other outdoor sports. That became almost impossible—but I have learned to do things I thought were impossible. I ride a bicycle, swim, and I can still hunt—I just walk a little slower than I used to. Now that my body is built back up again, I am feeling great. I work forty hours a week and am going to summer school at college. I enjoy fishing and swimming on the weekends and plan other activities through the week.

C106MA: Cancer of Both Lungs

This thirty-eight-year-old female had a right modified radical mastectomy in December of 1972. The post-operative diagnosis was infiltrating ductal carcinoma [cancer] of the right breast and metastatic carcinoma in three of the axillary [under arm] lymph nodes. Examination of the lymphatic system failed to reveal any lymphadenopathy. She had a normal bone scan and normal metastatic bone survey.

A January 9, 1973, letter from the radiologist, to whom this patient was referred, stated in part:

> I feel this patient is an excellent candidate for post-operative radiotherapy. Clinically, it ap-

> pears that younger women with breast cancer seem to suffer a more virulent course despite pathological grading. For this reason, I would be more inclined to be moderately aggressive in treatment planning and plan on treating the internal mammary, paraclavicular, and axillary apex areas as well as the chest wall to a tumor dose of 4500 rads in a five week period utilizing $Cobalt^{60}$. Possible complications and side effects of radiotherapy, including skin changes, esophagitis [inflammation of the esophagus], mediastinal and apical pulmonary scarring [lung damage], have been gone over with the patient and her husband.

The patient completed the suggested course of radiation therapy. The radiologist and the local doctor were both confident that the patient would continue to do well.

Two and one-half years later, cancer had returned at the site of the previous radiation. The patient states the local doctors recommended extensive surgery on both lungs. She was told that this would result in permanent hospitalization and dependency on machines to do her breathing. (This is an *unconfirmed* recommendation. We *hope* the patient misunderstood her doctor!)

The patient refused the recommended treatment and came to the Richardson Clinic for metabolic therapy. She stated that her local doctor had told her on July 27, 1975, that she had two months to live.

Metabolic treatment began August 7, 1975. The general health of this patient at the first visit was poor. She was pale, weak, and had difficulty breathing. She had a frequent productive cough. The sputum was green and streaked with blood. Significant hematology findings were lactic acid dehydrogenase 275 mu/ml and transaminase SGO of 54 mu/ml (lab normals, 7-40). Bio-assay tests were as follows: (1) August 7, 1975, 27.5, (2) August 28, 1975, 22.7, (3) October 24, 1975, 19.9.[1]

---

[1]See appendix for normals.

Patient reported on November 11, 1975, three months after beginning metabolic therapy, that she felt better than she had in the entire past year. She was still coughing in the morning on arising, but very little the rest of the day. The cough no longer produced green, blood-streaked sputum. Patient stated she could even run short distances.

Since that date, the patient has continued to adhere to her metabolic regimen of Laetrile, other vitamins, the special diet, and enzymes. Her response has been excellent and, at the time of this writing, her cancer appears to be controlled. She experiences no pain or other symptoms and carries on a normal daily routine.

B138I: Metastatic Cancer of the Lung, Previous Cancer of the Breast

In November of 1972, at the age of forty-nine, this woman had a radical mastectomy followed by twenty-four cobalt treatments for her cancer of the breast.

Six months later, chest X-rays showed a shadow on the lung. A biopsy was suggested but refused. The probable consequences of ignoring the situation were explained to the patient. Mrs. B. explained to her doctor, however, that her plan was to use Laetrile, because her sister was on Laetrile and (in the patient's words) "doing great." Mrs. B. said the doctor thought she was "crazy" for wanting to go on B_{17}.

The patient has been on metabolic therapy since 1972. She states she is strict about her diet and careful about taking all the recommended vitamins.

The shadow is still on the lung, but it has not grown and no longer appears suspicious of malignancy.

The patient contacted the Richardson Clinic in January, 1977. This period represents a three-and-one-half-year remission of probable cancer of the lung. The patient has had no treatment except Laetrile for the lung lesion.

CANCER OF THE ALIMENTARY TRACT AND MAJOR DIGESTIVE GLANDS

Case Histories Include: Stomach, Colon, Rectum, Anus, Liver, and Pancreas

The death rate of patients with cancer of the colon, rectum or anus who choose orthodox therapy and who do not use Laetrile *is second only to cancer of the lung.*[1] *More than 98 out of every 100 patients who have cancer of the pancreas and choose orthodox therapy will be dead in five years.*[2] *More than 99 out of every 100 patients with cancer of the liver are dead five years following orthodox treatment.*[3] *The following Laetrile case histories should be read with these facts in mind.*

S111E: Inoperable Cancer of the Rectum with Metastases to the Lung

This woman was admitted to State University Hospital, Upstate Medical Center, Syracuse, New York, on May 29, 1975. The history and operative report reads in part as follows:

> This patient is a sixty-four year old woman who was admitted to the hospital with an ad-

---

[1]*Clinical Oncology for Medical Students and Physicians, op. cit.,* p. 129.
[2]*Ibid,* p. 145.
[3]*Ibid,* p. 148.

mission diagnosis of carcinoma [cancer] of the rectum (established on recto-sigmoidoscopy with biopsy). The patient's current symptoms were those of a presence of local mass associated with symptoms of bleeding and tenesmus along with associated symptoms of early partial distal large bowel obstruction. . . .

Examination showed the patient to be an intact young appearing sixty-four year old woman whose physical findings were confined to examination of a rectum where digital examination disclosed the presence of a mass beginning 7 cms. cephalad to the anal verge [about 2.75 inches past the anal opening]. The mass appeared fixed and was attached to the posterior and lateral parietes. . . .

Barium enema demonstrated the presence of carcinoma of the rectum along with diverticulosis. . . . Chest X-ray showed evidence of metastases to both lung fields. . . . Alkaline phosphatase was normal. . . .

The patient was taken to the OR [operating room] where, despite the fixed appearance of the lesion with typical apple-core defect, she was explored in the hopes that a palliative resection [surgery to relieve the problem without curing it] could be performed. . . . At operation, it was discovered that, in addition to known pulmonary [lung] metastases, the patient possessed a large fixed, non-resectable [non-removable] carcinoma of the rectum.

Procedure was terminated by establishing a matured end-sigmoid colostomy through a stab wound and a mucocele through the distal operative wound. . . .

She understands the significance of her diagnosis and the extent of her disease and will be followed in my office and undoubtedly be placed on a course of chemotherapy.

The doctor just quoted is saying that before surgery the patient had cancer in both lungs and in her rectum, and after rectal surgery she still had cancer of the rectum because they could not remove it. All they could do was by-pass the cancer and bring her colon out through a hole in her abdomen (a colostomy) so she could have bowel movements. No attempt was made to remove the cancer of the lungs.

Let us now look at the "significance of her diagnosis" from the point of view of one highly respected surgeon. John H. Morton, M.D., Professor of Surgery, Department of Surgery, Member of the Clinical Cancer Training Committee, University of Rochester, School of Medicine and Dentistry, Rochester, New York:

> Gastrointestinal neoplasms [cancers] are mainly of surgical interest since the radiosensitivity of normal gut is high and most adenocarcinomas are radioresistant, producing an unfavorable radiotherapeutic ratio. . . .
>
> Colostomy for incurable rectal lesions is rarely palliative; such lesions should be removed by abdominoperineal resection when feasible whether or not cure is anticipated. . . .
>
> Chemotherapy in the author's [John Morton, M.D.,] experience has rarely been beneficial in metastatic colon cancer. The following statements have, however, appeared in the literature.
>
>> "Progressive, symptomatic, disseminated colon carcinoma can be palliated to some degree in about 20% of the patients with 5-fluorouracil. . . . "Objective responders show prolonged survival (20 months vs 10 months mean survival for non-responders)."[1]

Now, what all this means is (1) radiation generally does more harm to the healthy gut than to the cancerous part of the gut, (2) surgery is the treatment of choice, and it cannot be expected to do much good if the surgeon can't get all the cancer, (3) chemotherapy, in his opinion, rarely does anyone any good. Some doctors, however, think it might help one patient in five—at least a little bit. Some other doctors think you'll

---

[1]*Clinical Oncology for Medical Students and Physicians, op. cit.*, pp. 133, 134.

be dead in less than two years if you do just great, and you'll be dead in less than a year if you don't do so great.

When those of us who have looked into Laetrile say that patients, in general, are turning to it as a last resort this is the kind of situation about which we are speaking. This woman submitted to surgery, the "treatment of choice." Then she decided to try Laetrile and metabolic therapy to see if it could help her body defend itself againet impending death. Chemotherapy was refused.

Mrs. E's decision meant she had to make a 4,800-mile round trip from New York.

This patient began metabolic therapy, including Laetrile, on August 14, 1975. Her alkaline phosphatase before starting metabolic therapy was 92 mu/ml (normal, 30-85 mu/ml). It had been normal before surgery.

The patient states that X-rays taken in March, 1976, seven months after starting metabolic therapy, showed improvement in the lungs and the X-rays taken in December, 1976, showed no cancer at all in the lungs. She said that her local doctor, who knows she is on Laetrile, says it is probably just a "general remission," and she describes him as "typical of AMA doctors who refuse to acknowledge or even to condescend to accept the existence of Vitamin B_{17}."

The patient was telephoned in January, 1977, and said at that time, "For a patient who was only supposed to live a month [following the May, 1975, surgery] I'm not doing bad." Her voice was strong. She is leading an active life nearly two years following the initial diagnosis of inoperable cancer. She has had no radiation and no chemotherapy.

R159RX: Cancer of the Colon with Metastases to Lymph Nodes and Liver

This fifty-year-old man had a history of audible bowel sounds and abdominal cramps for three months prior to a barium enema examination on April 14,

1975, which revealed a 6-cm. (about 2.5 inches) filling defect at the junction of the descending and sigmoid colon.

Surgery was performed on April 22, 1975. The surgery report read in part as follows:

> The patient was found to have a tennis ball sized mass at the junction of the descending and sigmoid colon. The lesion penetrated entirely through the wall and there were several enlarged lymph nodes in the mesosigmoid colon at the site of multiple metastases. Although there were no other peritoneal metastases, the liver was filled with nodules of various size, measuring from 1 to 5 cm. in diameter in both the right and particularly, the left lobe of the liver. . . . [The tumor and a portion of apparently healthy colon were removed. Total length was 18 cm., or about 7 inches.] An end-to-end colostomy was then carried out. . . Postoperative diagnosis: Carcinoma of the colon with regional lymph node metastases and multiple hepatic [liver] metastases. Partial colectomy with end-to-end colostomy.

The pathology report dated April 22, 1975, states in part:

> *Microscopic Description:*
> The tumor is made up of bizarre colonic-type glands which are penetrating through the wall of the colon. In some places, they are fairly well differentiated. They arise from the surface, they invade lymphatics. Three of the six regional lymph nodes contain metastases.
> *Diagnosis:*
> Moderately well differentiated adenocarcinoma [cancer] of the colon, extending entirely through the wall and metastatic to three of the six mesenteric lymph nodes.

This patient came to the Richardson Clinic within a week following surgery and began metabolic therapy for the liver metastases. This was in April, 1975. At the time of this writing, patient has been symptom-free for nearly two years, and the only post-operative treatment he has received is Laetrile and metabolic therapy.

Patients whose cancer of the liver cannot be removed usually die within six months after the diagnosis is made.[1]

R168MS: Cancer of the Sigmoid Colon with Lymph Node Metastases and Extension into Mesenteric Fat

This sixty-six-year-old woman sought medical attention in June, 1975, because of a change in bowel habits. During the previous four months her stools had become reduced in circumference. She had also experienced lower abdominal cramping and some nausea but no vomiting.

There is a strong history of cancer in the family. One sister had cancer of the abdomen, one had leukemia, one had cancer of the brain, and one had lymphosarcoma.

Prior to the patient's admission for surgery, she had had multiple biopsies of the rectosigmoid (intestinal) lesion, barium enema, and sigmoidoscopy (visual examination of the inside of the bowel by instrument), all of which confirmed the diagnosis of cancer.

A portion of the sigmoid colon measuring 12.5 cm. (about 5 inches) was removed, and the remaining colon was sewn back together. The patient does not have a colostomy.

The pathology report from Mercy Hospital, Sacramento, California, dated June 24, 1975, states in part:

> *Microscopic Description:*
>
> Sections of the colon reveal the abrupt disruption of the colonic mucosa by infiltrative malignant neoplasm [cancer] variously composd of irregular glandular structures and solid sheets of cells which in the central position of the neo-

---

[1]*Clinical Oncology for Medical Students and Physicians, op. cit.,* p. 148.

plasm totally replace the muscularis and extend into the pericolic fat. . . . Extensive infiltration about the arteries is identified and neoplasm is found within vascular spaces which appear to be lymphatics, although special stains will be obtained to exclude venous invasion which may be present in at least one area. Eleven regional lymph nodes show metastatic malignant neoplasm involving one node. Perineural extension into the mesenteric fat is identified as well.

Special stains demonstrate elastic tissue in the walls of vascular spaces described above:
Diagnosis:
Segment of sigmoid colon showing:
(A) Extensively infiltrating poorly to partly differentiated adenocarcinoma [cancer] with extention into pericolic fat [fat around the outside of the colon].
(B) Metastatic malignant neoplasm [cancer] involving one of eleven regional lymph nodes.

Discharge summary dated July 2, 1975. States in part:

> Dr. C. [name omitted] saw her in consultation because of pericolic fat involvement and the metastasis to one node and he feels that chemotherapy was indicated which she has begun now. . . . She is discharged on Vistaril because she had nausea following 5-FU.

5-FU literature states that it is effective in the palliation (not cure) of "carefully selected patients who are considered incurable by surgery or other means. . . . Fluorouracil [5-FU] is a highly toxic drug with a narrow margin of safety."[1]

This sixty-six-year-old Catholic nun described her situation at that time in a letter to Blue Shield of California, which had refused to pay for her metabolic therapy. She felt it was "discriminatory" for them to pay for 5-FU, a palliative medication which made

---

[1]Literature enclosed with the drug by the manufacturer, Roche.

her sick, and not for metabolic therapy which made her feel well. The three-page typewritten letter reads in part:

> After my surgery in June of 1975, chemotherapy was recommended. I tried it and was not able to tolerate the medicine, since it made me very ill, depleted my energy, and made it difficult and even impossible to accomplish my work. I had to discontinue the chemotherapy.
>
> Fortunately, I heard of Metabolic Therapy which is a non-toxic, energy-building, disease-resistant treatment. I have been receiving this treatment for about three months with very beneficial results.
>
> These results are as follows:
>
> a. An increase of energy, enabling me to accomplish some work without tiring excessively.
> b. An upward trend in feelings of physical, emotional, and psychological well-being, with confidence that further treatment will maintain this upward trend.
> c. Confidence in the good effects of the therapy and in the professional competence of Dr. Richardson.
>
> Therefore, my right to choose a therapy that is good for me rather than one that is harmful (to me) should be allowed without discrimination. . . .
>
> Treatment with vitamins and minerals as well as food substances such as glucose is frequently administered to patients in hospitals as a means of building up the body to attain health. Medicare pays for these medicines when ordered by a qualified physician. . . .
>
> It is ironic that you have paid the maximum amount for the chemotherapy (5-FU) I received which caused me so much discomfort, yet you refuse to pay for treatment which has helped me.

This patient came to the Richardson Clinic on July 21, 1975. This was about four weeks following surgery. She had had three injections of 5-FU and then abandoned chemotherapy. Blood chemistry at the beginning of metabolic therapy revealed alkaline phosphatase 109 mu/ml (lab normals, 30-85), transaminase SGO 42 mu/ml (lab normals, 7-40), white blood cells 4.0 TH/cu.mm. (normals, 5-10 TH/cu.mm), red blood cells 3.8 mil/cu.mm (normals, for females, 4.0 to 5.5 mil/cu.mm).

She had 20 consecutive 9 gm. Laetrile injections I.V. and then gradually reduced doses of injectable Laetrile supplemented with oral Laetrile. She also received pancreas enzyme plus additional vitamins and minerals.

Her initial Bio-assay was 18.6 on July 24, 1975. Other Bio-assays were (1) 10-17-75, 14.8, (2) 3-20-76, 15.2 mg./1 (3) 5-15-76, 14.8 mg./1 (4) 9-10-76, 21.8 mg./1.

The patient stated in a letter received April 4, 1976, that for the first six months of treatment she was "almost 100% faithful to diet and vitamin supplements." Originally, it appears from her correspondence, she must have stayed with her family and later returned to her religious community.

She finds it difficult to maintain her diet within the confines of "institutional cooking," just as many business people who must travel away from home are challenged to maintain a vegetarian regimen while having only the restaurant or airline menus available to them. It takes real determination for the cancer victim, just as it does for the diabetic, and in both cases there cannot be too much emphasis on the value of the diet.

This patient's last contact with the clinic was January 17, 1977. At that time—one and one-half years following the incomplete removal of her cancer, her disease appeared to be satisfactorily controlled. She was experiencing no pain or other symptoms indicating cancer growth, and was able to lead an entirely normal and active life.

S163E: Cancer of the Sigmoid Colon

This patient was forty-nine years old at the time her symptoms began in the summer of 1963. She was troubled with persistent diarrhea. Sigmoidoscopy revealed a tumor, and the surgeon was insistent that the patient have surgery.

This woman decided to have a course of Laetrile prior to surgery in order to contain the cancer. This was administered by the late Byron Krebs, M.D., of San Francisco. (We do not have a record of the dosage. In general, however, the amount of Laetrile routinely administered was much less in the early 1960's than in the 1970's.)

The patient entered Kaiser Hospital in Oakland, California, and had a section of her colon removed on December 18, 1963. The surgery report states:

> *Final Diagnosis:*
> Adenocarcinoma of the colon arising in a villous adenoma.
> *Summary:*
> This forty-nine year old white female has been evaluated in the outpatient department with findings of a mass biopsied with findings of villous papilloma. . . .
>
> At exploration on December 18, 1963, a bulky tumor mass was noted in the mid-sigmoid colon involving a major portion of the circumference of the bowel with considerable surrounding edema. . . . Standard anterior sigmoid colon resection was carried out and the pathologic diagnosis report revealed adenocarcinoma of the colon arising in a villous adenoma with three of six lymph nodes showing replacement of normal tissue with tumor . . . there was invasion of mucosal and muscularis layers. . . .

The patient states that her husband was told by the surgeon that they had not been able to remove all the cancerous growth and she would need additional surgery in six months to a year.

She returned to Dr. Byron Krebs, and continued Laetrile injections twice a week for two years and what she describes as "a maintenance program at home."

The medical secretary of the Kaiser Hospital

record room states in a letter dated June 5, 1975, "the patient was last seen at our facility in December, 1970, at which time sigmoidoscopy to the hilt was negative [no evidence of cancer]."

Following the death of Dr. Byron Krebs, this woman became a patient at the Richardson Clinic. Although she has not been adhering closely to the prescribed maintenance levels of Laetrile recently, it is worth noting, that she is still alive and well *thirteen years* following surgery which left cancer remaining in her body. She has not had any radiation or chemotherapy.

L142N: Cancer of the Rectum

This woman was seventy-two years old when she came to the Richardson Clinic in January, 1975.

Prior to December, 1974, she had had a long history of good health, with no surgery or serious illness. In December she felt a small lump at the anal opening when she was inserting a rectal suppository.

Mrs. L. was examined by her local doctor and subsequently had a biopsy of the lump. Physical exam showed "an upper canal posterior tumor infiltrating up into the mucosa . . . , plus palpable posterior metastasis. Metastatic nodes, one at about two to three centimeters above the tumor, and another at about three centimeters above the node." Pathology reports stated the cancer was "infiltrating anaplastic squamous cell carcinoma."

As the patient was recovering in her room, she states, she overheard the doctor tell another doctor that she was, "too old to bother salvaging." At this point the patient, who never in her life had been a drinker, decided she would simply go home and drink herself to death since she could not be "salvaged." Upon leaving the hospital she stopped by a liquor store, and, having concluded that sherry would be the most lady-like alcohol with which to commit suicide, proceeded to purchase a case.

Mrs. L. was found two weeks later by her landlady, considerably the worse for having made a sincere, but fortunately unsuccessful, attempt to "sherry herself to death." It was at this point that a friend suggested Laetrile therapy as a substantially superior alternative.

She began metabolic therapy including Laetrile January 22, 1975. A notation on the chart one week later says the patient states she "never felt better in her life."

She has continued to stay on the diet and vitamin program. She has had no surgery, radiation, or chemotherapy. She continues to be symptom-free and in excellent health nearly two years after her initial diagnosis.

Lest someone assume this lady imagined the doctor's comment, it seems appropriate to include a portion of the letter her physician wrote to another doctor, a copy of which is in the patient's file. After briefly describing the patient's history and the biopsy results (pathology diagnosis), he stated:

> She certainly needs local suppression, but did not yet get X-rays of the chest, liver scan, chemistries, etc. . . . After 5-6,000 rads, maybe I might consider abdominoperineal resection—although mortalities in her age group barely make it pay in terms of salvage.[!]

She *was* "salvaged" and without radiation or a permanent colostomy.

H132I: Cancer of the Colon

On April 5, 1973, two polyps were removed from the sigmoid of this fifty-nine-year-old female patient. The pathology report from Sutter Community Hospital in Sacramento, California, dated April 6, 1973, concludes, "Diagnosis: *Sigmoid polyps received as three pieces: one piece showing adenomatous polyp. Two pieces showing moderately well differentiated adenocarcinoma.*"

Mrs. H's local doctor urged immediate surgery, explaining to the patient that she possibly would have a colostomy following surgery. She sought the opinion of two other M.D.'s in the Sacramento area—one of whom was a proctologist—and both doctors concurred that immediate surgery was essential to save the patient's life.

The patient states that she was acquainted with people who had been successfully treated for various kinds of cancer with vitamin therapy. She investigated and decided this was what she wanted to do.

Mrs. H. began vitamin therapy April 26, 1973. She gained back the ten pounds she had lost and states she experienced a sense of well-being and increased energy soon after beginning her treatments. Subsequent sigmoidoscopy revealed the rectum and sigmoid to be completely free of any cancer.

The patient states she follows the diet "100%" and continues to take the vitamin supplements.

She has had no recurrence in the three years since she was told to have surgery or die. She has had no surgery, no radiation, and no chemotherapy.

L129G: Cancer of the Colon, Previous Cancer of the Uterus and Breast

This forty-nine-year-old woman had her uterus removed in 1965. She states she was told it was not cancer but that she was a very lucky person because they "got it all."(!)

In May of 1971 the patient discovered a lump on her left breast. She did not seek treatment until September, 1971. By this time, the nipple had retracted, and the tumor was affixed to the chest wall. Biopsy performed October 1, 1971, at San Leandro Hospital, San Leandro, California, was positive. The patient was advised she had six months to a year to live, assuming she had cobalt treatments, which she did. She describes herself as looking like a "basted turkey" and feeling very weak. The tumor still could be felt at the conclusion of cobalt therapy. She states the treated area is still numb to the touch—four and one-half years later.

In April, 1972, the patient began to have the

same "tired all the time" feeling which preceded her other medical problems, so she went to Mexico for diet and vitamin treatments, which did *not* include Laetrile.

The patient states she began to have difficulty having bowel movements, her abdomen was swollen, and then she developed severe pain associated with bowel movements during March and April, 1973. She returned to her local doctor who, after a diagnostic work-up, stated she must have surgery. Part of the colon surrounding the tumor was removed, and the remainder of the colon reconnected in May, 1973. The surgery report states:

> There were numerous areas of studding throughout the mesentery of the entire small bowel, of large lymph nodes and succulent glands seen all along the colon mesentery as well as from this widespread metastatic involvement. [Eden Hospital, Castro Valley, California.]

Chemotherapy was recommended but refused by the patient. According to Mrs. G., her doctor advised her that without chemotherapy she had only two weeks to two months to live.

The patient, at this point, returned to her program of vegetarian diet and vitamins and also came to the Richardson Clinic for Laetrile injections. At the completion of her initial course of therapy, she had fully recovered from her surgery, had no more pain, had gained weight, and was returning rapidly to normal health.

Over three years have now passed since she was told she had only a few weeks to live. She continues on metabolic therapy at a maintenance level, and her cancer appears to be controlled. In a letter to the Richardson Clinic dated March 25, 1976, the patient states she feels good, can put in a full day's work, and continues to have favorable check-ups from her local doctor, who is dumfounded by her continued good health.

P131B: Cancer of the Colon

June 4, 1975, this sixty-five-year-old female was found to have a cyst in her rectum. Pathology report was positive for cancer.

The patient was admitted to the local hospital for five days for further studies to establish the probable extent of the cancer. Then, without consultation with the patient, surgery was scheduled.

The patient and her husband were both startled by the arbitrary attitude of the local doctor. The doctor advised the patient that if it were his wife, he would not let her leave the hospital without the benefit of surgery. The patient was advised that forgoing surgery would be a drastic mistake and probably would cost her life. Mrs. P. said she was greatly disturbed by her physical condition and "to add to the confusion the doctor became very hostile."

The patient came to the Richardson clinic for metabolic therapy in July, 1975. She states in a letter dated April 6, 1976:

> I was very weak when I started his [Dr. Richardson's] treatment and also had some pain. Very soon I was able to attend meetings and do my housework and am now living a normal life. The growth has diminished in size and I now have normal bowel movements. I am following my diet closely and am feeling better.

It is one and one-half years since her diagnosis. She has had no surgery, no radiation, and no chemotherapy. The tumor has receded, and the patient is symptom-free.

C120C: Inoperable Cancer of the Rectum

This fifty-three-year-old male had a ten-year history of colitis. He felt the problem was getting worse in April of 1974 and went to his local doctor. He advised the doctor that he had lost thirty pounds in forty-five days, but was told it was only colitis.

In August of 1974, he was found unconscious in

his home and rushed to the Veteran's Hospital. Emergency surgery was performed, and a colostomy was created. Cancer was found at that time, but it was felt that the patient was too weak to survive removal of the tumor from the rectum. Plans were made for him to go home and try to gain strength to withstand the additional surgery.

The tumor of the rectum was removed in November, 1974, but the doctors decided to delay closing the colostomy. The patient was readmitted for the third time in February, 1975, to have the colostomy closed. Examination revealed, however, that there had been extensive regrowth of cancer, that it was inoperable, and closure of the colostomy was out of the question because he would be unable to have a bowel movement.

According to the patient, he was advised to "Go home, make out a will, put your affairs in order, and then come back to the hospital. We'll try to make you as comfortable as possible during the little time you have left."

The story of what followed is related here in the patient's own words on November 29, 1975.

> When I took my leave of absence from the hospital, I was so weak I could hardly walk. I grabbed onto things as I went down the hall to the bathroom, which was very often. At night I was taking the sleeping pills and the pain pills the doctor suggested. That made getting down the hall every fifteen minutes even harder.
>
> I talked with my sisters, and we all cried about my hopeless situation. Then I called friends in Los Angeles to say goodby, and they said I should try Laetrile. That was about the third time someone had said Laetrile to me. I decided, since I had nothing to lose, why not try it?
>
> At this point, I had been reduced to eating baby food and broth. I was so weak I had to be driven to the clinic for that first visit [February 20, 1975].
>
> I gained eight pounds during the first two weeks of treatment. I began to think there was

hope. I decided to go to the race track near the clinic and watch the horses. I'm a betting man, and I know horses. I was careful, and I finally made enough money to pay off my loans, pay for my treatment, and have enough money left to go to Hawaii in the summer.

While in Hawaii, I had the Veteran's Hospital proctoscope me. They said the tumor was twenty per cent smaller than the Palo Alto Veteran's Hospital reported five months earlier. That made me feel so damn good I came back to California by way of Alaska. I tell you, I really have hope. I may be living on borrowed time, but I'm living free, not al tied down in some grey hospital room.

There is little that could be said from a medical point of view that would add much to the above information.

This patient's hemotology studies were all within normal limits. His bio-assay tests were as follows: (1) February 20, 1975, 25.6, (2) March 19, 1975, 22.8, (3) April 9, 1975, 19.2 (4) July 24, 1975, 18.5.[1]

Mr. C's chances for long-term survival are slim. By his own admission, however, the year following Laetrile therapy was quite different from the original, grim predictions.

L167MX: Cancer of the Head of the Pancreas

This seventy-two-year-old woman had suffered from indigestion for a number of years. In March, 1975, her indigestion became worse. Examination in April, 1975, indicated possible obstruction of the common bile duct.

She was examined again in August, 1975. Hospital summary states she had a bilirubin of 7mg.%, alkaline phosphatase of 605 (lab normals, 40-85), SGOT 510, sedimentation rate of 30. Echogram did not show a tumor in the pancreas.

---

[1]See appendix for normals.

It was decided, however, to perform surgery for what was thought to be a gall bladder problem.

Surgery was performed on September 6, 1975. The diagnosis before operation was, "Obstructive jaundice secondary to extrahepatic biliary obstruction."

The diagnosis after surgery was, "Carcinoma [cancer] of the head of the pancreas." A procedure known as a Whipple operation was performed. Part of the patient's stomach, duodenum, the head of the pancreas, the common bile duct, and the gallbladder were removed.

The surgery report states in part:

> . . . At this point [in the operation] it was noted that the mass palpable in the head of the pancreas was intimately adherent to the posterior wall of the portal vein. It appeared grossly that the lesion was a carcinoma of the head of the pancreas. By very tedious and slow dissection, the adherence of the tumor mass to the portal vein [vein to the liver] was dissected free, and this was completed without further trauma to the vessel.
>
> It should be noted that the tumor was divided in the posterior aspects to accomplish this, and a small portion of tumor was left in situ as the procedure was completed.

Following the incomplete removal of this woman's cancer of the pancreas, the tissues removed were submitted for pathology diagnosis. The pathology report dated September 8, 1975, concludes:

> *Diagnosis:*
> Portion of stomach, duodenum, and attached pancreas showing:
> (A) Well-differentiated infiltrating adenocarcinoma [cancer] large duct type, involving head of the pancreas with extention to the surgical margins.
> (B) Single lymph node with metastic carcinoma.

Other body parts which were removed did not contain cancer, but were in some cases inflamed or contained cysts.

The patient states that following surgery she inquired how long she might have to live and was told, "You might live two weeks, two months, or two years. We do not know." The suggestion of two-year survival under the circumstances of the operation seems to be closer to psychotherapy than statistical reality, for, in truth, the average patient with advanced cancer of the pancreas lives only six months following surgery.

According to James T. Adams, M.D., of the University of Rochester:

> Essentially, the five year cure rate is less than two per cent. In one of the few irradiation studies reported, the average survival for the advanced patient not irradiated was 6.1 versus 6.6 months for the patient irradiated.[1]

This patient was not offered radiation or chemotherapy.

The patient states:

> I can well remember the hopelessness I experienced after being told by my surgeon, who had discovered the cancer of the pancreas, that I had, "two weeks, two months, or two years" to live, probably because he was unable to remove the entire cancerous growth. My internist said there was really nothing he could do. . . .
>
> A relative suggested Laetrile, which I had never heard of but, as there was nothing to lose, I started treatment.

This woman came to the Richardson Clinic and began metabolic therapy including Laetrile on October 21, 1975. Blood studies were within normal limits.

---

[1]*Clinical Oncology for Medical Students and Physicians, op. cit.*, p. 145.

Minerals were balanced based on hair analysis. Her first Bio-assay was 26.2. She received twenty 9 gm. I.V. injections of Laetrile supplemented later with oral Laetrile tablets. Her most recent Bio-assay on November 2, 1976, was 19.6 mg./1.

She was last seen at the Richardson Clinic on January 31, 1977. At that time it had been eighteen months since her surgery and fifteen months since beginning metabolic therapy, which she had continued at a maintenance level. Her diarrhea has gone, she had no pain, her appetite had returned, and she reported that she felt strong and healthy. Her disease appears to be under control.

F115L: Inoperable Cancer of the Liver, Previous Cancer of the Breast

This patient had a right radical mastectomy in September, 1969, which was followed by radiation therapy.

Nearly five years later, in June, 1974, during a routine physical exam, the patient was found to have an enlarged liver. Subsequent liver biopsy was negative. Laparotomy was performed and the diagnosis of metastatic cancer (of the breast) to the liver was made.

The tumor could not be completely removed, and following surgery the patient was placed on Methosarb. This had to be discontinued because of adverse effects on her blood chemistry.

Later, she was started on 5-FU. This required her carrying around a pump so the 5-FU could be continuously pumped into her liver artery. The artery became blocked, and by mid-October of 1974 all chemotherapy was discontinued.

The patient states that after the failure of an attempt to re-start the 5-FU she felt "deeply depressed."

In early December, 1974, a friend told her about a symposium being held near her home. The subject of the talk would be Laetrile. This woman had been given up by orthodox medicine, so she went to hear what had to be said about Laetrile. Based on the information at the symposium she decided to try it.

She was sixty years old when she came to the clinic. She describes her first shot of Laetrile, received on December 26, 1974, as her "day after Christmas present." She said, "My spirits rose, and I again had hope that I might achieve a remission of sorts; but in light of previous failures, I was hesitant to let my hopes soar too high."

When this patient visited the clinic in January, 1977, she was a very young-looking sixty-two-year-old. It had been two years since she had received any treatment other than Laetrile and metabolic therapy.

She stated that she had been very faithful to the diet. During the first two years following the start of treatment she had eaten meat only twice—once on Thanksgiving and once on Christmas. She was continuing her maintenance level of Laetrile, other vitamins, and enzymes, and is leading a completely normal life.

Under orthodox therapy, cancer of the liver is almost certain death. James T. Adams, M.D., of the University of Rochester states "the course of the disease [liver cancer] is rapid if the tumor is nonresectable [cannot be removed]. Most patients die within six months after the diagnosis is made."[1]

A139DJ: Metastatic Cancer of the Liver, Primary Cancer of the Colon

This sixty-three-year-old male noted bright red bleeding in his stools in October, 1974. This continued intermittently, so he consulted his local doctor in March, 1975. An 8-cm. (about 3 inches) tumor was discovered in the rectum, and the biopsy revealed it to be cancer (invasive adenocarcinoma of the colon, grade III).

The surgery report dated March 20, 1975, from

---

[1]*Clinical Oncology for Medical Students and Physicians, op. cit.,* p. 148.

Permien General Hospital in Andrews, Texas, reads in part as follows:

> *Postoperative Diagnosis:* Carcinoma of the rectum metastatic to regional nodes and to the liver.
> *Operation Performed:* Abdominal perineal resection with formation of permanent colostomy.
> *Tissue Removed:* Distal sigmoid colon and rectum.
> *Pathology Found:* To my great sorrow, Doug, a really fine, fine, guy, has at least eight or nine palpable nodules, unfortunately involving both lobes of the liver, very typical of cancer. There seems to be a node or two over on the right side of the colon just beyond the peritoneum, too. I did elect, in this gentleman's case, however, to go ahead with the formal abdoninal perineal resection, because Doug has never been sick in his life, and I just don't see that he would tolerate mucous and blood from his rectum on a prolonged basis at all.

Mr. A. came to the Richardson Clinic to begin metabolic therapy on July 29, 1975. He has had no radiation or chemotherapy for the cancer not removed by surgery.

In a letter to the Richardson Clinic dated April, 1976, Mr. A. stated that he was maintaining his weight and that his color and appetite had returned. He was continuing on vitamin therapy and adhering to the recommended diet.

Since that time, he has continued to have routine check-ups from his local doctor, and as of March, 1976, there had been no indication that the nodules on the liver were enlarging. Our last contact was one year following colon surgery and identification of inoperable cancer of the liver. At that time the patient was well and leading a normal life.

As we were going to press a letter dated January 19, 1977, was received from the patient's wife. It stated in part:

I want you to know how much we, Doug and I, appreciate all you have done and are doing, to help people to get the necessary nutrition to help their bodies overcome the deficiencies that exist. . . .

Doug began his vitamin therapy in July of 1975. His color is good and he has maintained his weight. We have other friends who have not been on this therapy and have not done as well.

We feel that Doug's condition is due to the fact that he has been on vitamins, including Laetrile and B_{15}.

Our prayers are with you in this battle. Thank you again for what you are doing.

This represents nearly a two-year survival of a patient with inoperable cancer of the liver.

CANCER OF THE FEMALE GENITALS

Case Histories Include: Cancer of the Uterus, Cervix, Vulva, Vagina, and Positive Pap Smears

Orthodoxy claims that only one out of every five patients with cancer confined to the cervix will be dead in five years.[1] *Statistics could not be located for cancer of the cervix which had penetrated surrounding tissue, but they probably would show a mortality rate of at least two times that of a restricted site. One of every three patients with cancer of the uterus* who do not use Laetrile *but choose orthodox therapy instead will be dead in five years.*[2] *Cancer of the ovaries, when treated by orthodox methods, accounts for a greater number of deaths than all other genital cancers combined. Two out of every three patients with cancer of the ovaries* who do not choose Laetrile *but choose orthodox therapy instead will be dead in five years. Over one-half of all patients with cancer of the vagina who submit to orthodox treatment are dead within eighteen months.*[3] *Keep these facts in mind when reading the following Laetrile case histories.*

---

[1]*Clinical Oncology for Medical Students and Physicians, op. cit.*, p. 166.
[2]*Ibid*, p. 172.
[3]*Ibid*, pp. 174, 181, 183.

W166I: Cancer of the Uterus and Cervix

This sixty-two-year-old woman has a remarkable history of change in Pap smear and tissue studies in just six months. She had had routine physical exams, including normal Pap smears, until March, 1976, at which time the Pap smear report stated, "Atypical cells present. Possibly adeno-origin."

On May 13, 1976, a biopsy was performed and the pathology report read in part as follows:

> *Microscopic Diagnosis: Endo biopsy of endometrium showing mucin secreting adenocarcinoma* [*cancer*]. Although it is possible that this is a mucin secreting adenocarcinoma arising in the endometrium or endocervix, a metastatic lesion must also be considered.

On May 21, 1976, there was a second evaluation by another pathologist, who, on the basis of the tissue studies, confirmed the diagnosis of cancer.

This woman had not proceeded with the recommended treatment, and finally on June 8, 1976, three months after the initial positive Pap smear, she received a letter from her doctor at Kaiser Permanente Medical Group in Oakland, California, which read in part as follows:

> The purpose of this letter is to review your medical situation and to state our opinion in regard to the treatment of your condition. . . .
>
> The pathology report of the tissue obtained was adenocarcinoma of the endometrium. Subsequently, additional tissue was obtained from the endocervical canal and this, too, showed adenocarcinoma of the endometrium. . . . My conclusion was that you had endometrial carcinoma [cancer] of the uterus with extention to the cervix. . . .
>
> At that time, I, too, [in addition to another medical doctor] advised you that the appropriate treatment for this condition would be hysterectomy with postoperative irradiation with Cobalt

> to the side pelvis externally and radium to the vaginal vault.

The letter continued pointing out the dangers of not seeking the suggested treatment and advising the patient that if she would not accept the recommended treatment they could not be responsible for the outcome of her disease.

This woman came to the Richardson Clinic to begin metabolic therapy including Laetrile on June 14, 1976. Blood studies were within normal. She received 9 gms. of Laetrile I.V. daily for twenty days and then the I.V. dosage was gradually reduced and supplemented with Laetrile tablets on the days she did not recieve shots. According to the patient, she accepted the vegetarian diet and followed it without allowing herself any exceptions.

She had a Pap smear on September 29, 1976, about three months following the beginning of treatment. The findings were, "Class I—negative." No cancer was present.

Tissue pathology exam on December 17, 1976, was also negative for cancer.

The patient wrote the Richardson Clinic November 12, 1976. The letter stated in part as follows:

> The advice of the surgeons left me in a state of emotional shock. I felt after seeing them that I had to prepare for impending death.
>
> My first visit to the clinic of Doctor Richardson changed my mind. I had the good luck of meeting a young woman from Santa Barbara, California, already in the waiting room who had been his patient for over two years. She looked healthy, radiant, and full of energy. She had recovered from cancer of the breast through vitamin therapy. . . .
>
> [This sixty-two-year-old woman continues her summary]. I lost weight during the first six weeks of the diet—something I had always wanted. I felt a little weak during the first week, and did less jogging than the three miles I usually

do each morning. But, I worked in my hard, stressful, and demanding job without any interruption and without anyone noticing any change. As a matter of fact, to this day, I've had no more than three days vacation all summer and fall.

The most important fact to me is that I could continued my normal life in all its forms during my treatment, without any absence from work, without pain or other problems. I consider myself healthier now than before, less strained.

L152L: Cancer of the Ovary

Mrs. L., a sixty-one-year-old woman, went to her local doctor on November 5, 1975, because of a brownish discharge from her vagina. Examination revealed a mass on the right side of her pelvis.

The patient was hospitalized for exploratory surgery. On November 17, 1975, her uterus, both fallopian tubes and both ovaries were removed. The frozen section on the right ovary showed adenocarcinoma (cancer). The final pathology diagnosis, from Dameron Hospital, Stockton, California, was "clear cell carcinoma—('mesonephroma') stage I-C."

In addition to the cancer of the ovary, "floating" cancer cells were identified in the peritoneal fluid.

When the patient went back to her local doctor for a six-week check-up, he felt a small lump near the line of the surgical incision.

The patient stated that her local doctor was insistent that she have radiation. When advised that she simply could not afford it, he said she should at least have chemotherapy, which would not be so expensive. Mrs. L. stated that her doctor warned her that without radiation or chemotherapy, she would have no more than a year to live.

Approximately a month following surgery, Mrs. L. came to the Richardson Clinic for metabolic therapy, including Laetrile. She has responded favorably and, despite her doctor's dire predictions, continues to enjoy good health and to lead a normal life without pain or the disability from radiation or chemotherapy.

M158SX: Cancer of the Ovary

This woman was seventy-one years old when she was admitted as an emergency patient in June, 1973. She had had progressive abdominal pain and swelling. Also, this patient had a severe cough and, in addition, she was unable to have a bowel movement.

Surgery report stated in part:

> A massive right ovarian, lobulated and degenerative tumor was found, there was a solid, necrosing, degenerating carcinoma of the ovary. There were multiple abdonimal ovarian intestinal adhesions and a large amount, [4,000 cc.] of acetic fluid was present. The right ovarian tumor . . . had to be dissected from the right ureter . . . the pathology reports of the tumor showed adenocarcinoma of the right ovary with extensive hemorrhage, necrosis and cystic degeneration.

The other pertinent laboratory and X-ray findings were: (1) Chest X-ray: bilateral pulmonary congestion, (2) Barium enema: multiple diverticula of the colon, (3) IVP: ureters normal on both sides but incomplete drainage of the right renal collecting system, (4) Bone scan: suggestive of a neoplastic (cancer) process of D6, dorsal vertebra, (5) Admitting blood count: 11.9 gm. hemoglobin, 32,300 WBC's, 80 segs. Alkaline phosphatase was 3.3, (6) Class III cells were found in the fluid removed from the abdomen.

Because of the nature of the surgery (having to cut around the ureter leaving cancer tissue behind) and the suggestion on the X-ray of cancer metastasis to the spine (D6 vertebra), further treatment was recommended following surgery. The July, 1973, discharge summary concludes:

> It was felt pelvic irradiation with cobalt would be in order and subsequent chemotherapy to be instituted as patient was evaluated during the course of time. The family was consulted as to the very guarded prognosis.

The patient's daughter said that the family was advised the patient would probably not live three months. The daughter stated:

> Even though I refused, the doctor set up a cobalt appointment for mother. We cancelled. Her weight prior to her illness was 140 pounds. In the hospital she went down to 125 pounds and by the time we arrived at the Richardson Clinic her weight was down to 110 pounds.

Mrs. S. came to the Richardson Clinic and began metabolic therapy in August, 1973. Within a month, she had gained fifteen pounds and returned to her pre-illness level of strength.

Mrs. S. has remained on Laetrile and the other recommended vitamins and minerals and continues to follow the recommended diet.

At the time of publication, this seventy-three-year-old woman—who was given three months to live—has now extended that grim prediction to three and one-half years. This is truly impressive in view of the fact that she had an incompletely removed ovarian carcinoma with metastasis to the spine. Nevertheless, her latest contact with the Richardson Clinic revealed that she feels strong enough to fly back and forth across the United States by herself to visit family and friends. She continues to be symptom-free, and it appears that her disease is controlled.

M122T: Cancer of the Cervix, Stage I

This fifty-five-year-old patient began "spotting" from the cervix in mid-January, 1975. Subsequent exam at Kaiser Hospital in Oakland, California, revealed cancer of the cervix, Stage I.

Surgery was planned for March 10, 1975. The physician noted on February 22, 1975: "Patient is going to have cancer surgery; uterine involvement; radical hysterectomy. Mrs. M. has not told her husband because she is concerned about his heart condition."

Mrs. M. explained later that she decided not to go through with the surgery because she had seen her mother die of cancer after having had surgery and radiation. She had heard her mother say before her death that, if she had to do it again, she would never have submitted to surgery; rather she would have "lived with the lump."

The patient began metabolic therapy March 4, 1975, at the Richardson Clinic. (She sought out the Clinic after hearing Laetrile discussed on the Tom Snyder TV Talk Show.)

In a letter to Mrs. M. dated March 27, 1975, the gynecologist at Kaiser Hospital expressed his concern about her failing to keep her surgical appointment in these words:

> This is to inform you that you have an invasive carcinoma of the cervix. You have failed to keep two admission dates for surgery for therapy of this carcinoma.
>
> I have been unable to reach you by telephone.
>
> You are strongly urged to contact this office to arrange or follow-up and treatment.

The patient states that she was also advised that she would be, "dead in three months" if she did not have surgery or radiation.

In spite of these admonitions, the patient continued with metabolic therapy and refused surgery or radiation. Pathology report from a Pap smear taken March 18, 1975, revealed: "Class I negative. No atypical cells present [no cancer]." That was only fourteen days after starting metabolic therapy.

Notation from Dr. Richardson at the Richardson Clinic on September 25, 1975, (after pelvic exam of Mrs. M.) states: "Patient still bleeds easily. No visible tumor." This was seven months following the diagnosis of cancer of the cervix, Stage I.

Mrs. M. stated in a letter to the Clinic dated March 13, 1976 (one year after her initial diagnosis):

I decided to start Laetrile because in my opinion the FDA did not offer any logical argument against it.

I started Laetrile treatment on March 4, 1975. I cancelled my original surgery date and moved it to March 21, 1975. However, after three weeks on Laetrile, I felt so energetic I cancelled surgery again. The two doctors called me at home and at work. They talked to my husband [whom the patient had not wanted to be informed about her diagnosis]. One doctor told me the tumor would kill me in three months if I did not have surgery.

I followed the diet with very few exceptions. In my first year I have had no meat, no coffee, no liquor, and no dairy products. I take the Laetrile and other vitamin supplements every day. I still take one 10cc. shot [3 gms.] of Laetrile every week.

I have not been back to Kaiser for an examination since I feel well and healthy. I work every day at my job, and am active in my community.

I have not developed any other lumps. I have not lost weight. I feel strong. This is sufficient proof to me that my cancer is under control.

When my doctor [the one who wanted her to have surgery] asked me if I knew how painful death from cancer would be, I said yes I knew. My mother had breast cancer. She was butchered and burned and died a slow and painful death. We had to keep her arm in ice packs twenty-four hours a day because of cobalt burns. My mother was not helped or saved. That is precisely why I rejected surgery and radiation.

Mrs. M. is still a healthy, active woman as of January, 1977, two years following diagnosis of cancer of the cervix. She has been appointed to the Community Development Agency of one of northern California's large counties. She has been involved in planning rehabilitation of older homes in her community. One of her current goals is to work for the establishment of a community center in her home town. She also paints in her "spare" time.

B133L: Cancer of the Cervix

This twenty-eight-year-old woman went to her local doctor in November, 1975, complaining of severe pain in the area of the cervix, a heavy vaginal discharge, and extreme tiredness. The Pap smear was Class III. The patient was advised to come in for another Pap smear, colposcopy (visualization of the cervix), and a biopsy. The patient had only the second Pap smear.

Finally, at the urging of her family, she went to the University of California Medical Clinic in San Francisco, California, and had a third Pap smear and, this time, a colposcopy and a biopsy. The biopsy was positive for cancer of the cervix. Pathology diagnosis of the January 28, 1976, biopsy was, "squamous cell carcinoma in situ, cervix." Surgery was advised strongly.

The patient chose instead to come to the Richardson Clinic in January, 1976, for metabolic therapy, including Laetrile. She states in a letter received in April, 1976, "I have improved quickly both physically and emotionally. The pain is gone, the discharge is gone, and so is the tiredness. I am no longer afraid of cancer."

The patient went back to the same doctor at the University of California Medical Clinic for a re-examination in April, 1976. The patient states, that upon seeing her, the gynecologist (who knew she was on vitamin therapy) laughed and said, "I'll bet you think it's gone, don't you?"

It *was* gone. The doctor could find nothing suggesting cancer. Even the biopsy site had healed. Another Pap smear was taken. The patient states the doctor left the room immediately after taking the Pap smear and did not want to discuss the vitamin therapy at all.

Material from this woman's cervix described as "white epithelium peeled off cervix" was submitted for pathology evaluation on April 14, 1976. The pathology diagnosis was, "strips of dyplastic epithelium (white epithelium peeled off cervix)." No Pap smear classification was given and no indication of cancer was found. This is a change of tissue from obvious cancer to no observable cancer in just three months.

The patient was last seen at the Richardson Clinic in January, 1977. At that time, there was every indication that her cancer had been controlled successfully.

A101AJ: Pap Smear Class V

Mrs. A, a forty-one-year-old female, went to her local doctor for a routine physical; the Pap smear taken at the time, May 24, 1973, was class IV+. The pathologist report stated: "Many groups of abnormal squamous cells are noted that are highly suspicious of malignancy. Advise IMMEDIATE repeat smear for cytologic confirmation."

One week later, May 30, 1973, the repeat Pap smear was class V for carcinoma in situ. The pathologist stated: "Many groups of cells suggestive of malignancy noted. Advise D&C and conization."

In March, 1974, she again was examined by her local doctor, and the Pap smear was again class V. The doctor reported:

> A repeat Pap test by Dr. [name omitted] showed the same result as did a biopsy. There was no doubt, whatsoever, that this was a very small carcinoma with minimal tissue invasion.

This patient was opposed to any surgery and, after considerable delay, went to the Richardson Clinic for metabolic therapy. This was begun on March 10, 1975.

Pap smear pathology report of April 1, 1975, (three weeks after starting metabolic therapy) stated: "Class II atypical, cells present consistent with benign [non-cancer], cellular changes."

Upon conclusion of the initial course of metabolic therapy, she had a repeat smear. Pap smear pathology report of May 28, 1975, stated: "Class 1, no atypical cells present." There was no longer any evidence of cancer.

In a letter dated March 3, 1976, the patient stated she had been to her local doctor "about three months ago" and that he told her everything looked good. She further stated that the Pap smear taken at that time was Class 1 (no cancer).

There are two final thoughts that come to mind in this case. One is that some women apparently can have identified cancer and not progress as rapidly as is generally assumed to be the course in cancer of the cervix. The second is more subtle. This woman very likely also would have had a Class 1 Pap smear following a course of radiation therapy. Extensive radiation to the cervix and nearby tissue, however, can produce a permanent irritation of the vaginal wall, making marital relations out of the question. Though this might not be of vital concern to her radiologist, it certainly would to the patient and her husband.

K124M: Class IV + Pap Smear

This patient was forty-nine years old at the time of her first Class IV+ (cancer cells present) positive Pap smear, which was performed in June, 1973. She had a cervical scraping, which was positive, and a positive zerogram. The doctor insisted that she have a hysterectomy, and her husband was strongly urging her to go along with the doctor's recommendations.

About this time, the patient states, "The wife of one of Doctor Richardson's patients was visiting her daughter who lives in my home town, Davenport [Iowa]. She was told about my report and made a special call to my home to tell me about vitamin therapy. She made the necessary arrangements and encouraged me to go. In her words, 'What have you got to lose?' "

The family was so against her decision that they refused to co-operate in any way. She took a bus and came out to California alone.

She had her first Class I (normal, no cancer

cells) negative Pap smear July 12, 1973, only *nine days* after starting on metabolic therapy.

The staff at the Richardson Clinic describe her crying for joy, and after her happy tears she obtained a photocopy of the Pap smear, autographed it, "With kindest regards"—and mailed it back to the family. There was a happy reunion in Davenport at the conclusion of the initial course of therapy.

Routine Pap smears during the subsequent three years have continued to be negative. The patient says she does not stay on the diet but does continue most of the vitamins and eats eight apricot kernels a day.

Her family doctor can offer no explanation for the negative Pap smears. The patient states he flatly refuses to discuss Laetrile, saying the only possible answer is, "You are one in a million that a scraping cured."

P162N: Pap Smear, Malignant [Cancer] Cells Present

At the age of thirty-four, this woman had a Pap smear during a routine physical examination at Mason Clinic in Seattle, Washington. The Pap smear, taken on September 9, 1974, was positive. The report stated, "many malignant [cancer] squamous cells."

An appointment was made for a cold knife conization [removal of a cone of tissuc] and biopsy study of the material removed from the cervix. The patient states that she was advised due to the presence of cancer cells in Pap smear material that she would most likely need a hysterectomy.

This woman was familiar with Laetrile and metabolic therapy and decided to cancel the cold knife conization, much to the distress of her local doctor. She arrived at the Richardson Clinic on October 10, 1974, and began the usual series of twenty 9 gm. I.V. shots of Laetrile. Mineral intake was balanced in accordance with her hair analysis. Blood studies were essentially normal, with the exception of the transaminase SGO, which was 175 mu/mu (lab normals, 7-40).

Repeat blood studies on January 7, 1975, showed

the transaminase SGO had risen to 206 mu/ml. A Pap smear was repeated on January 7, 1975. Pathology report stated, "Class III, atypical cells present consistent with marked squamous dysplasia."

This patient's response to metabolic therapy was much slower than some of the other cases in this section on Pap smear response. She is included, however, to emphasize the variation in time of patients' responses to metabolic therapy.

The Pap smears are listed in chronological order:

9-9-74	Many malignant [cancer] cells.
1-7-75	Class III, atypical cells present consistent with marked squamous dysplasia.
11-18-75	Class IV, abnormal cells present suggestive of carcinoma.
3-15-76	Class III, moderate dysplasia [abnormal cells that are not positively cancer].
11-3-76	Class I, negative [normal, no cancer cells present].

This woman has had no treatment for her cancer of the cervix except metabolic therapy including Laetrile.

She wrote the following on the back of her 1976 Christmas card to Dr. Richardson and his wife, Julie.

> Thanks for the good news. . . . Please use my case in your book with my deepest gratitude.

She included a photograph of herself and her three little girls. She is the picture of radiant good health.

CANCER OF THE MALE GENITALS

Case Histories Include Cancer of the Prostate

Cancer of the prostate is the most prevelant cancer in men over fifty years of age. Under orthodox therapy it is the second most common site of cancer causing death in the male.[1] *Virtually 100% of patients will be impotent following surgery.*[2] *Once metastasis is present nearly 100% of patients choosing orthodox therapy will be dead by the end of the third year.*[3] *Read the following case histories with the above facts in mind.*

P107J: Inoperable Cancer of the Prostate

This man was sixty-one years old when he went to Kaiser Hospital in Sacramento, California, in August of 1973. His complaint was pain in the pubic area.

Numerous exams were performed, including a biopsy of both lobes of the prostate gland. The pathology diagnosis was "well differentiated adenocarcinoma" (cancer) of both the right and left lobes of the prostate.

A bone scan was performed in September, 1973.

---

[1]*Clinical Oncology for Medical Students and Physicians, op. cit.*, p. 203.
[2]*Ibid*, p. 206.
[3]*Ibid*, p. 206.

The report stated "Impression: Abnormal bone scan demonstrating an increased uptake of tracer by the right anterior-superior iliac spine [part of the hip bone]. No other abnormalities noted."

Urology consultation in October, 1973, stated in part:

> Bone scan shows a hot spot over the anterior-superior iliac spine. This plus elevated bone marrow acid phosphatase removes him from the operative group. . . . We will follow him regularly and, should the bone metastases increase, or bone pain develop, or serum acid phosphatase increase, or local extention of tumor occur, or obstructive symptoms develop, we will then begin stilbestrol [female hormone] daily, with or without orchiectomy [removal of testicles].

The patient states the doctors told him that surgery would only increase his suffering and that they were going to wait until his symptoms were no longer tolerable before attempting the only procedures available. He says he was grateful for their honesty.

The patient states further that he asked the doctor "how much time" he had and was told he had one plus on a scale of four.

The patient related in a letter to the Richardson Clinic what the next few weeks were like for him:

> My condition following the testing became rapidly worse. I was in constant, unrelenting pain, my body jerked in spasms, there was some rectal bleeding, and I became so weak I could hardly rise from a chair and walk.
>
> At this time I learned from friends where I could get Laetrile treatment.
>
> My wife drove the car, the one and one-half hour drive to the San Francisco Bay area where I received my first injection of Laetrile, October 25, 1973. I was too weak to drive, in fact I passed out in the car both going to and returning from these first daily treatments.
>
> Improvement was apparent within ten days

> and in about thirty days I was driving the car myself. I was again looking forward to each new sunrise with anticipation of some pleasure in being alive.

The patient was concerned at first that the Kaiser Hospital doctors would refuse to give him check-ups when advised he was taking Laetrile, but they have continued to see him and are pleased with his obvious good health.

This patient was interviewed at length on October 29, 1975, two years following his diagnosis of inoperable cancer of the prostate. His eyes and skin were clear, and his conversation animated. He proudly showed the nurse some scratches on his right arm and announced they were from chopping wood. He stated the doctors had given him about a year to live, (this was two years later) and then he concluded:

> I figure I'll renew the lease for another year. You know, I go back to my other doctors about every three months just so they will see how well I'm doing and know they don't have all the tools available to them.
>
> I am the sixth of eleven brothers and sisters to get cancer.

The patient has been essentially symptom-free now for over three years. He states, "I feel so good it bothers my wife because I can go all day and get along on four hours' sleep, and she can't keep up with me." This statement is from a man who three and one-half years ago was too weak to drive himself to the clinic.

H151W: Cancer of the Prostate

This man was sixty-nine years old when he first developed symptoms which his local doctor considered to be an inflamed prostate gland. The symptoms began January, 1974, and he finally sought medical help on October 8, 1974. He did not improve much when treated with tetracycline.

Because of his failure to improve, his local doctor had him admitted to a hospital near his home in Stockton, California, for further tests. Cystoscope exam revealed a completely obstructing prostate. Both sides of the prostate were removed and the tissue was cancerous (well and poorly differentiated adenocarcinoma).

He was placed on Estradurin injections in the hospital and started on Estinyl tablets, 0.05 mg., one a day. These are female hormones which are considered to be useful in providing *temporary* control of the spread of cancer beyond the prostate.

A radiotherapist advised him to have X-ray to his chest to prevent female type breasts from developing due to the female hormones he would be receiving. The radiotherapist also advised a "full course" of radiotherapy to the lymph nodes of the pelvis. The patient's survey for metastases and his bone scan were negative.

The patient was against radiotherapy, explaining to the radiotherapist that he had seen someone with very poor response to cobalt and did not want the same for himself.

His acid phosphatase was elevated 3.1 units over a normal of 2.

In a letter to the Richardson Clinic, dated January 14, 1975, the local doctor stated:

> I hope Mr. H. has a very slow growing tumor and that it would be sensitive to estrogen control. He seems to be not a candidate for either radiotherapy for cure nor orchidectomy [removal of testes] at the present time due to his emotional state. If he could stay on the estrogen tablets once a day, I think all would be well for the time being.

The patient not only refused radiation and what is referred to as "therapeutic" removal of his testes but also stopped taking the estrogen tablets after only twelve days.

Mr. H. came to the Richardson Clinic to start metabolic therapy including Laetrile on January 3, 1975.

He says he has been faithful to the vitamin program, and about fifty per cent of the time he stays on the diet.

Mr. H. wrote the Richardson Clinic, March, 1976, and stated:

> As you know, what was left of my tumor has disappeared. My general health is better than before surgery. I have much more energy and no aches and pains. I'm a seventy-one year old man and work on a ranch almost as hard as I did twenty years ago.

This man remains symptom-free two years after his initial diagnosis and the incomplete removal of prostate cancer.

B144J: Cancer of the Prostate

This man was sixty-two years old at the time he first sought treatment for a prostate problem. That was in the fall of 1968.

Diagnosis of cancer was made by his local doctor. The patient stated he was advised that if he did not agree to surgery or radiation, he would not live long. The patient described the tumor as being about the size of "a bar of soap."

Mr. B. originally sought the services of another physician in the San Francisco area. He went on a strict vegetarian diet at that time and still maintains the same dietary regimen. He received injections of Laetrile every four days from January of 1969 to January of 1970.

Mr. B. has been seen at the Richardson Clinic intermittently since September, 1971.

As of February, 1976, Mr. B. is seventy years old. He still works his farm. His days are full of activity *eight years* after being told that without treatment he had only months to live.

The only treatment he has received is metabolic therapy including Laetrile.

A140R: Cancer of the Prostate, Probable Cancer of the Liver

Mr. A. had had intermittent difficulty urinating for two years prior to October 13, 1975, at which time he went to his local doctor because he was completely unable to urinate.

Examination revealed an enlarged prostate. Biopsy was positive for cancer. Lymphangiograms indicated the cancer had spread to the adjacent lymph nodes.

Exploratory surgery, October 20, 1975, showed the patient had widespread involvement of the lymph nodes and cancer of the liver. The extent of the cancer made surgical removal impossible, and neither radiation nor chemotherapy was recommended.

The patient stated he was sent to Stanford University, Palo Alto, California, for further evaluation and that their recommendation was to withhold the use of female hormone therapy until the patient felt worse. The reason for waiting is that female hormone therapy appears to slow down the cancer growth for a limited time only.

The patient explained his reaction to the limited therapy available this way. "They told me they could do nothing more. I don't know how to explain my feeling. I never felt it would get the best of me." The patient's daughter gave him a book on Laetrile, and, encouraged by what he read, he decided to try it.

Mr. A.'s first appointment at the Richardson Clinic was November 19, 1975. At the time he was weak from the abdominal surgery and still had difficulty urinating. Six weeks after starting metabolic therapy he had returned to work full time; he no longer had difficulty urinating, and stated he "felt great."

The prostate has decreased somewhat in size. The only therapy the patient has received (following incomplete surgical removal of his cancer) is metabolic therapy. He continues to work full time and to enjoy life in good health.

B109WJ: Cancer of the Prostate

This seventy-five-year-old man had a biospy of his prostate in February, 1973. The biopsy revealed cancer. He refused surgery or radiation. Lymphangiograms taken at that time were negative for metastasis.

This patient came to the Richardson Clinic for metabolic therapy July 12, 1973. An initial physical exam revealed a small hardened mass on the right lobe of the prostate. Approximately five and one-half weeks after beginning metabolic therapy, physical exam showed that the mass had decreased.

In October, 1973, the patient stated he had just returned from a vacation during which time he had "out golfed" his son. He said, "If I felt any better, I wouldn't know how to act."

This patient visited the Richardson Clinic on January 16, 1974. During that visit he stated he had had a left herniorraphy. Recovering had been uneventful except for mild left leg pain. The patient stated that his surgeon found the prostatic tumor to be very small with no visible signs of metastasis.

In a letter to the Richardson Clinic dated March 3, 1976, (three years after he had been advised he had cancer) he summarized his experience in part as follows:

> I had seen my mother dying of cancer. She had both surgery and radiation, which probably extended her life for a year or so, but she suffered more from the treatment than from the cancer itself. It was then that I had made up my mind that if I ever had a cancer, I would rather just let nature take its course than go through all that. So, I did nothing for the first couple of months, but I got to feeling so bad I went back to Dr. [name omitted] and had him give me a prescription for the female hormones [previously suggested]. I took these for perhaps a month. Be-

sides feeling no better otherwise, the hormones made me feel like I had been castrated, sort of in limbo between a man and a woman, and I began to grow breasts.

By now I was getting so I could only work a couple hours and then I would have to rest or go to bed for a time. [The patient then describes medical consultations regarding radiation, and his subsequent decision to come to the Richardson Clinic.]

I saw you [Dr. Richardson] in July, 1973. You had so many patients waiting in your outer office that day, it was several hours before you could get to me. It was time well spent because the reports I got from a number of your other patients out there astounded me. I made up my mind then and there to cancel my radiation appointment. . . .

In the middle of August, my wife and I went back to Pennsylvania to visit a daughter of mine and her husband. . . . I felt so peppy, I amazed them that a man in his 70's could show the stamina I seem to have at golf, dancing, etc. . . .

I am now 75; I am still working and enjoying it. Of course, I am delighted with what vitamin and nutritional therapy have done for me.

Of all your patients, I am sure there is not one who stays on the diet more strictly than I do. As a matter of fact, the more I am on it the more I enjoy it.

One final observation. It seems to me that, if vitamin therapy and the use of Laetrile in cancer therapy were quackery, there would be no end of complaints from patients and their relatives. There is no cry from your patients, only from the purveyors of radiation, chemotherapy and surgery; and what have they got to boast about? If the record of Laetrile were half as bad as theirs, they would be burning you at the stake. They accuse the Laetrile doctors of "ripping off" the public to the tune of forty million dollars a year with a useless remedy. I have my own opinon about who, if anybody, is doing the ripping off, and not to the tune of forty million. More like sixteen billion.

L123A: Cancer of the Prostate

This sixty-two-year-old man went to his local doctor for a routine check-up in November, 1974. The physician felt a lump on the prostate.

The patient was subsequently referred to a urologist, who recommended a biopsy. The biopsy report dated February 28, 1975, stated the diagnosis as "moderately differentiated prostatic carcinoma [cancer]."

In a letter dated March 7, 1975, the urologist described Mr. L's situation:

> Since Mr. L's [name omitted] perineal needle biopsy showed carcinoma, and since rectal palpation indicated that it had already extended beyond the prostatic capsule (or at least involved it), I have advised him to have radiation therapy after a thorough metastatic workup.

A subsequent letter dated March 28, 1975, revealed the patient's situation to be even more dire.

> Unfortunately, the lymphangiogram showed positive nodes and the KUB suggested ileal metastases. This precludes radiation therapy.
>
> I talked with Mr. L [name omitted] and his son in the office. Since the hormonal therapy, which would be the proper treatment, has a limited and predetermined duration of effectiveness, I don't think that we need start it until he has symptoms or some findings which indicate progression of the tumor. Accordingly, I'm going to check him in three months and keep an eye on him. He seemed to take the thing psychologically better than I expected, after all his troubles.

Among the other "troubles" that this gentleman had was the fact that he was fired from his job as soon as they found out he had cancer.

Mr. L. stated, "This proposal not to have any help shocked me, and my mental state was beyond description." It was at this point that he turned to vitamin therapy as a last resort.

Metabolic therapy was begun April 8, 1975. After two months, the patient began to feel improvement in his general health. In a letter dated August 25, 1975, the consulting urologist stated, "Mr. L. seems to be holding his own well."

Examination of the prostate on November 17, 1975 (seven months following commencement of metabolic therapy), revealed no sign of tumefaction.

Mr. L. stated again in December, 1976, (one and one-half years after being diagnosed as inoperable and non-radiatable) that he was feeeling good and that his cancer apparently had been successfully controlled.

K114M: Cancer of the Prostate

In July, 1974, this sixty-six-year-old man had a routine physical exam. His family doctor found a lump on the prostate and referred him to a urologist.

The urologist had him admitted to Mercy Hospital in Carmichael, California, for a needle biopsy. The report, dated July 29, 1974, stated, "prostatic tissue showing adenocarcinoma." Radiation therapy was recommended but was refused by the patient because of the possible side effects of sterility and impotency.

The patient decided to try metabolic therapy, which was begun August 26, 1974. Approximately one year later, July 16, 1975, physical examination failed to show any tumefaction whatsoever.

At the time of this writing, over two and one-half years following biopsy, the patient was symptom-free and in good health.

B108C: Cancer of the Prostate

This sixty-eight-year-old male had a biopsy of the prostate on May 29, 1975, at Washoe Medical Center, Reno, Nevada. The pathology report stated in part, "Left prostatic needle biopsy . . . focus of well differentiated adenocarcinoma." He was given a choice of surgery or radiation.

The patient chose, instead, to come to the Richardson Clinic for metabolic therapy. At the time of his first visit, he was essentially symptom-free except for a palpable tumor in the left lobe of the prostate. Metabolic therapy was begun on July 8, 1975.

After an examination, on July 31, 1975, the physician stated: "There really is no sign of residual tumefaction." The patient remains on his diet and medications. He continues to be free of symptoms and in good health.

CANCER OF THE URINARY TRACT

Case Histories Include Cancer of the Bladder

Between 57 and 90 out of every 100 patients with cancer of the bladder who do not choose Laetrile *but choose orthodox treatment instead will be dead within five years.*[1] *Orthodox treatment has many serious and pairful side effects. It is important to consider these facts while reading the following Laetrile case histories.*

E148M: Cancer of the Bladder, Previous Cancer of the Cervix

Mrs. E. was forty-eight years old in September, 1972, when she was diagnosed as having "poorly differentiated invasive endocervical carcinoma." Uterine curettings revealed adenocanthoma. Bilateral inguinal node biopsies, September 15, 1972, were negative.

An examination of the cervix revealed it to be hard and irregular and largely replaced by necrotic tumor. The radiologist stated, "I think there is medial parametrial involvement." (This means he thought the cancer had also gone into the tissue and smooth muscle around the uterus.)

In a letter dated September 22, 1972, the patient's physician—the radiologist from St. Joseph's Hospital in Stockton, California, explained:

---

[1]*Clinical Oncology for Medical Students and Physicians, op. cit.,* p. 202.

> I plan 3500 rads whole pelvis radiation. I may possibly give an additional 500 rads to the left parametrial area. This will then probably be followed by 5000 to 5500 mg hours in two separate radium application.
>
> She understands that complications may occur in spite of precautions. I also told her that chances were reasonably good, but that a cure could in no way be guaranteed. She understands these issues quite well I think.

The patient was treated with $cobalt^{60}$ and radium implant therapy from September through December, 1972, for her Stage II cervical cancer.

Two years later, July, 1974, the patient was referred by her gynecologist to a urologist in Stockton, California, because of blood in her urine.

The bladder had a lesion which, in the opinion of the urologist, was cancer. No treatment was recommended according to the patient—perhaps because of the extensive radiation the area had already received. The patient states she was given a few months, at most, to live.

Mrs. E., a widow and a grandmother, was "putting her affairs in order" when a salesman came to her door with a multi-volume children's Bible set. The patient was impressed with the series and wanted to purchase it for her grandchildren. She explained to the salesman she could not purchase the Bibles despite her wish to do so because there was very little chance she would be alive long enough to complete the time payments.

Mrs. E. told the salesman that she was dying of cancer. He asked her if she had heard of Laetrile, and when the patient said no, the salesman left and returned several hours later with books on Laetrile for Mrs. E. to read.

The material she read, combined with the hopelessness of her situation under orthodox therapy, led Mrs. E. to make an appointment at the Richardson Clinic and begin a course of metabolic therapy including Laetrile on August 7, 1974.

The patient responded beautifully, as is evidenced by the comments of her urologist in a letter to the Richardson Clinic dated November 19, 1975, (sixteen months after she had been pronounced terminal). The letter reads in part as follows:

> I saw Mrs. E. initially in referral from her gynecologist on July 15, 1974, concerning bladder irritative symptoms and gross hematuria of several days duration.
>
> Office cystourethroscopy [visualizing the inside of the bladder by instrument] on July 22, 1974, disclosed a fungating bleeding posterior urinary bladder floor lesion that had all the appearances of tumor extension, while she had a low capacity urinary bladder undoubtedly associated with some delayed radiation cystitis. . . . The lesion had the appearance of neoplasm in my sixteen years of experience.
>
> Mrs. E. returned on November 12, 1974, requesting repeat cystoscopy and at that time, the patient was having gross hematuria [blood in the urine] with a few clots each morning and had been receiving medication from you [i.e., Richardson Clinic] for approximately three months. . . .
>
> Mrs. E. returned on November 17, 1975, with a "tugging" type of discomfort in her mid-pelvic region. She had had no gross hematuria for approximately one year. Repeat cystourethroscopy showed no urinary bladder floor lesions at this time, although there was a whitish area where the original lesion had been and one could see the definite outline of same. It appeared to represent some type of smooth and glistening scar tissue. Repeat pelvic examination again demonstrated definite tenderness and even more vaginal stenosis [due to previous radiation]. A bimanual rectal examination failed to disclose exidence of masses beyond the area of the cervix and urinary bladder floor. . . .
>
> Needless to say, I was most happy with Mrs. E.'s current situation and wished her the best of luck.

B104G: Recurrent Cancer of the Bladder

This man was sixty-three years old at the time he first sought medical treatment for blood in his urine. In October, 1974, he was X-rayed, cystoscoped (viewing of the bladder), and the tumors in his bladder were removed. The pathology report identified the tissue as "papillary type transitional cell carcinoma of the bladder, grade I to II." The surgery report states approximately 8-10 gm. of tissue was removed.

Three weeks later, surgery was performed, and additional cancerous tumor was removed. The patient, an investment counselor who lives near St. Louis, Missouri, was strongly urged to have his bladder removed. He was unwilling to submit to this surgery, so radiation was scheduled.

He received 6500 rads of cobalt during a fifty-seven-day period between November 26, 1974, and January 15, 1975. During this time the patient described himself as weak, listless, subjected to intense abdominal cramping, and as passing clotted and fresh blood in his urine. Also, during this same period he had to be hospitalized because of acute urinary retention.

May, 1975, four months after the completion of radiation treatments, surgery was again required to remove more cancerous tumor.

In November, 1975, for the second time since the radiation therapy, it was necessary to remove additional cancerous tumors. At this point, the patient stated, "The doctor concluded at this time that I should be examined every ninety days. To me, this was an ominous sign, and I decided on vitamin therapy without further delay."

Mr. B. began metabolic therapy including Laetrile on January 15, 1976. He stated he has been conscientious about taking all the vitamins and has adhered strictly to the vegetarian diet. This is not an easy regimen for an individual who must eat frequently away from home.

Mr. B. was examined again by his local doctor on March 15, 1976, and the patient stated that three small clusters of grade II carcinoma were found. Eight months later he was examined again and advised that the cancer was no longer progressing.

It is important to restate the fact that, during the eleven months of "orthodox" therapy, five hospitalizations were required plus fifty-seven days of the out-patient treatment for cobalt therapy. Two of the surgeries were *subsequent* to the cobalt treatment.

During the twelve months of maintenance therapy on Laetrile, his only other medical expenses were for two cystoscopic exams from his local doctor.[1]

In a letter to the Richardson Clinic dated January 5, 1977 (one year following the beginning of metabolic therapy), Mr. B. concluded:

> I have been under your treatment and have followed your recommended diet for a year and, quite frankly, I have never felt better nor had more energy. I submitted to cystoscopic examination in late November, 1976, and there was no apparent cancer progress. I was discharged from the hospital in record time.
>
> I expect to continue your recommended treatment and diet for the remainder of my life, and we pray that nothing may happen to impede you in your work.

H143E: Cancer of the Bladder

This man was fifty-eight years old when he first began to develop cancerous bladder tumors in 1971. (He had a previous history of squamous cell carcinoma of the lip. It was resected in 1965.)

In August, 1971, Mr. H. began to pass blood in his urine. Subsequent examination revealed cancer of the bladder "Grade IV, Stage A transitional cell carcinoma." The tumors were removed, along with part of the bladder.

---

[1]The medical bills were vastly different under the two modalities (consensus medicine vs. metabolic therapy). Are there any insurance companies out there which would care to join our crusade for metabolic therapy?

His symptoms returned a year later. Admission history from St. Mary's Hospital in Reno, Nevada, dated June 22, 1973, states in part:

> The patient was seen initially by me in August, 1972, with gross hematuria [blood in the urine]. . . . The patient was scoped by me and was noted to have recurrence of tumor. This was resected. The pathology showed transition cell CA [cancer] Grade III to IV in multiple sites. He was brought back for one more resection, again Grade III CA . . . in addition . . . a prostate resection. . . . September, 1972, patient was noted to have microscopic foci of well differentiated adenocarcinoma . . . The patient completed his radiotherapy [5,400 rads] around February of this year [1973].

The fourth bladder surgery was performed on June 26, 1973 (four months following radiation). Multiple bladder biopsies were taken and then the two areas of cancer were fulgurated (burning of tissue by means of high frequency electric sparks). Pathology report stated the tissue received was "transitional carcinoma [cancer], Grade II."

November 19, 1973, the patient's bladder was again examined. Two areas of tumor were found. The patient's records from the Nevada hospital do not state what specifically was done about the tumors identified in November, 1973.

The patient again developed blood in the urine late in 1974. He states that the doctor advised him he could not receive any more radiation because he had already received the maximum allowable.

Apparently, the only thing that was done for the patient was to put him on Percodan for the pain. There was some question of inguinal gland involvement in cancer, and the patient also developed pain in his right hip. Lymphangiograms done at the time were inconclusive because of previous radiation to the area.

This man concluded that he had exhausted all possibilities with conventional therapy, so he turned to metabolic therapy including Laetrile. This was begun January 16, 1975.

Within two weeks he was no longer requiring the pain-killer Percodan, and instead of regularly passing large red clots of blood in his urine he was passing only occasional tiny clots, which he states were the size of a "match head."

The patient has continued on his maintenance dose of vitamins and, at the time of this report, was essentially symptom-free. This represents a two-year absence of bladder problems while on Laetrile. (A previous two-year period between August, 1971, and August, 1973, required four surgeries and 5,400 rads of radiation—at the conclusion of which the patient still had tumors of the bladder, blood in his urine, and the need for the pain-killer Percodan.)

A141JA: Cancer of the Bladder

This man was sixty-four years old at the time he went to his local doctor in October of 1974 because of discomfort in the area of the bladder. Physical examination revealed an enlarged prostate.

On October 21, 1974, the surgeon performed a transurethral removal of the prostate gland and a bladder tumor. Post-operative diagnosis was papillary carcinoma (cancer) of the urinary bladder and benign prostate hypertrophy (non-cancerous enlargement of the prostate gland).

Cystoscopic examination of the bladder was performed on February 18, 1975, and June 17, 1975. The physician's summary stated:

> The first tumor was posterior to the original resected area, and another small area was noted anteriorly at the bladder neck. These tumors had increased in size from February 18 to June 17 of this year.

Because this man had experienced a return of tumors following removal of the first cancer, he decided to seek metabolic treatment as an alternative to further surgery. He began metabolic therapy on July 22, 1975. Our last contact with this patient was in January, 1977, one and one-half years later. At that time he was maintaining his therapeutic program, was symptom-free, and it appeared his cancer was controlled.

C134CR: Cancer of the Bladder

This seventy-two-year-old woman has an extensive history of surgeries, most of which have been for cancer.

1). 1948—Removal of the uterus and ovaries, reason not clear to patient. Records not available.
2). 1959—Removal of left breast for cancer.
3). 1967—Bladder surgery: Polyp removal.
4). 1968—Colon surgery: Thirteen inches of malignant colon removed. Was told she might have five more years to live.
5). 1971—Bladder surgery.
6). 1973—Bladder surgery: Patient was told next surgery would require its removal.
7). June, 1975—Bladder surgery to repair damage from previous examination. Malignancy found. Patient was told it was inoperable. Radiation and chemotherapy were urged by the doctor. Both were refused by the patient.

Mrs. C., who is a practicing lawyer, reflected on her medical problems in this way.

> I felt whipped down by these continual operations, and wondered why, with all the expenditure of money for investigation, no cause of, or remedy for, cancer had ever been found. It seemed to me that the doctors were only removing symptoms; no one had any suggestions as to why the cancer continued to recur.

The patient states she heard about vitamin therapy through friends in Oakland, who suggested she contact Dr. Richardson. Vitamin therapy was begun in March of 1975. It will be noted that this was two months before the last discovery of cancer. That does not invalidate the case, however, for it took more than two months for that bladder cancer to develop, and the usual pattern for regression of any cancer (that is to say the lump itself) in the experience of this clinic, is that the regression is steady but slow. It should be emphasized, however, that the concern of the clinic is not the lump but the total physiological milieu of the patient. This is in stark contrast to the lump-oriented thinking of orthodoxy, which says it does not matter much how the patient looks or feels as long as something is done about the lump.

Mrs. C. had been on metabolic therapy for a year at the time of our last contact with her. She stated her life has "entirely changed." She has discussed the use of metabolic therapy with her local doctor, who continues to remain noncommittal. She stays on the diet faithfully, with the exception of variations necessary because she also has hypoglycemia. She continues to take the suggested supplements.

In a letter postmarked March 28, 1976, the patient commented on the impact of vitamin therapy and on the quality of her life in these words:

> There has been no need for further operations; I feel better than I did at the age of forty and I'm now seventy-two. I am a retired lawyer who now serves on numerous public and church commissions and committees; I do gardening on an acre and a quarter of lovely garden and orchard; I am an organist in a Rescue Mission Chapel; I travel extensively, and still give legal aid when called upon by clients or the local bar association.

And *that* is quite a schedule for a seventy-two-year-old lady with a long history of cancer!

CANCER OF THE SKIN

Case Histories Include Malignant Melanomas Only

Patients with malignant melanoma who do not use Laetrile *but use orthodox therapy instead have the following death rates depending on the extent of their lesions: (1) One out of every two patients with lesions at one site only will be dead in five years; (2) Of patients who have positive regional nodes, more than eight out of ten will be dead in five years; (3) Not one patient will be alive in five years among those who have lesions with distant metastases.*[1] *The following case histories should be read with these statistics in mind.*

A100WPX: Cancer of the Scalp, Cervical Spine, and Part of the Hip Bone (Amelanotic Melanoma With Metastasis)

This patient's symptoms began in June, 1972. The medical summary report, dated August 19, 1972, from the University of Oregon Medical Center described her thus:

> *Subjective:* This twenty year old student nurse was referred because of leg pains, unexplained neurologic symptoms, and elevated sedimentation rate. She had gradual increasing malaise, weakness, and weight loss for approxi-

[1]*Clinical Oncology for Medical Students and Physicians, op. cit.*, p. 225.

mately six months. . . . About one month before this admission [7-30-72], an occipital [back of the head] swelling was noted.

Objective: . . . Brain scan was normal, but showed intense radio active uptake in subcutaneous occipital area. [Total excisional] biopsy of scalp mass: Undifferentiated malignant tumor, origin unknown.

Hospital course: The documented sites of tumor involvement are scalp, cervical spine, and right acetabulum [part of the hip bone]. Though origin of tumor is unknown, a good possibility is amelanotic melanoma. . . .

The patient and her mother are aware of the malignancy and its poor prognosis. Despite her illness, this deeply religious patient maintained a cheerful outlook. . . .

[Discharge summary states:] Complete diagnosis of the tumor was impossible with various possibilities being listed as follows: (1) amelanotic melanoma; (2) Reticulum cell sarcoma; (3) histiocytoma, and (4) possible embryonal rhabdomyosarcoma.

Impression: Highly malignant anaplastic carcinoma [primitive cell cancer] of unknown cell type and primary presumed to be amelanotic melanoma [cancer of the skin, originating from a mole-like growth but lacking the typical mole coloring].

Within a week, there was a regrowth of the mass on her posterior scalp. There was great concern that fracture of the adjacent vertebrae would result in the patient being paralyzed from the neck down. During this time, September, 1972, the patient received radiotherapy, and the tumor mass almost completely disappeared.

At the same time, however, she developed severe back pain, and the radiotherapist felt there was evidence of metastasis in this area and began additional radiation. The patient was receiving Delaudid for pain.

By July 16, 1973, symptoms had returned, and

the hospital put her on MOPP regimen consisting of nitrogen mustard I.V., Vincristine I.V., Procarbazine, and Prednisone.

Patient had the usual reaction to I.V. nitrogen mustard with rather severe nausea and vomiting. Her pain continued as did complaints of generalized malaise, abdominal pain, sleeplessness, and constipation.

Notation on July 31, 1973, stated: "Patient is manifesting rather marked toxicity to her chemotherapeutic regimen. Therefore, she is not scheduled to receive any medication for the next two weeks."

The patient, who is a nurse, described the effect of chemotherapy in these words:

> My reaction to CCNU [an abrreviation for a currently used drug] each six weeks was one of dread. I spent twelve hours constantly vomiting, though sedated with Secobarbital and Compazine. I accepted it matter of factly, as I chose to continue my nursing education, and I knew no other treatment.
>
> CCNU continued until May, 1973, when I went out of remission. Recurrent back pain in the thoracic and lumbar area led to another week of radiation therapy.
>
> In June, 1973, I had several doses of Bleomycin to tide me over until my blood count was acceptable for the MOPP regimen [nitrogen *m*ustard; vincristine (*O*ncovin); *P*rocarbazine; and *P*rednisone] which started in late June.
>
> With this [MOPP] I felt awful all the time, lost all my gained weight, lost my appetite, and began having constipation problems. My mouth was sore. I could hardly eat and had no energy left.
>
> I returned home in early August [1973], as I could no longer continue school. I was told if I stopped chemotherapy I had only three weeks or so to live. My doctor in Roseburg, Oregon, followed me for one more week of drugs. Then, against his advice, I stopped.
>
> He was pessimistic about my future, but I felt the quality of my remaining days was more important than the quantity. I trusted the

> Lord would give me strength for whatever came up. I had no fear—only peace and contentment that at last the hell of the drugs was over.

This patient first came to the Richardson Clinic in September, 1973. She was so weak she needed her parents' help to walk into the clinic. As a result of her chemotherapy, she was bald, had no appetite, and had been bedridden. Her weight was 107 pounds.

Metabolic therapy was begun September 9, 1973. It was the patient's wish to be able to spend one more Christmas with her parents before she died. She did spend Christmas with her parents, but she did not die. In a letter dated March 22, 1976 (two and one-half years after being told she would live only two months), the patient describes her experiences during the first month of metabolic therapy.

> I had no more pain after three days on Laetrile [and the metabolic therapy regimen]. My energy and spunk had started to come back. I was able to go back to nursing school in late September full time with no trouble. . . . *With my return to health, I had to be careful of a resentment of typical cancer treatment, as I saw so many of its failings.*

The following observation was made following a medical exam at the University of Oregon Medical School dated April 22, 1974.

> In the spring of 1973 she was felt to have recurrent metastatic lesions to the thoracic and lumbar vertebrae and again underwent a course of radiation therapy. Since approximately August, 1973, the patient has refused further chemotherapy, but has continued to do well. At her last evaluation in February, 1974, in Chemotherapy Clinic, the lesion in the occipital region of her skull was felt to be decreasing in size and no new lesions could be identified.

She has continued on a vegetarian diet, with some exceptions, and metabolic therapy. In late 1974, the patient discussed with Doctor Richardson her wishes, and those of her husband, that they have a child. In September, 1975, after an uneventful, normal pregnancy, this young woman delivered a healthy baby girl.

She continues to be symptom-free as of our last contact with her in December of 1976—more than three years after her doctors told her she would be dead.

CANCER OF THE HEAD AND NECK

Case Histories Include: Cancer of the Nose, Tongue, Throat, Vocal Cords, and Tonsil

Three out of ever four patients with cancer of the tonsil and positive nodes who do not use Laetrile *but choose orthodox therapy instead will be dead within five years.*[1] *Two of every ten patients with cancer of the vocal cords who choose orthodox therapy will be dead in five years.*[2] *Those patients who do survive therapy for cancer of the face usually suffer extreme cosmetic deformities. The following case histories should be read with these facts in mind.*

P103MX: Cancer of the Lymph Glands in the Neck and Cancer of the Base of the Tongue

In April, 1964, at the age of thirty-seven, this woman detected an enlarged lymph gland on the side of her neck. Biopsy revealed "poorly differentiated squamous cell carcinoma." The patient had surgery—a left radical neck dissection for removal of all the lymph nodes—and, at the same time, the entire right side of her thyroid and part of the left side of the thyroid were removed. Later pathology exam of all thyroid tissues

---

[1]*Clinical Oncology, op. cit.,* p. 242.
[2]*Ibid,* p. 246.

showed "thyroiditis" [inflamed thyroid] but no evidence of cancer.

Several years later she had a non-cancerous tumor, a neurofibroma, removed. The surgery resulted in the paralysis of her left vocal chord, and also paralysis of her diaphragm.

Nine years later, in May, 1973, at the age of forty-six, she developed a lesion at the base of her tongue. Biopsy was positive. Pathology report revealed "poorly differentiated squamous cell carcinoma, transitional cell type." She was referred by her local hospital to Massachusetts General Hospital, Harvard Medical School.

Physical exam revealed an irregular mass 2 cm. by 2 cm. at the angle of the jaw. Examination of the mouth revealed an approximately 2 cm. by 3 cm. (¾ inch by 1¼ inches) mass at the base of the tongue on the left and "extending down into the vallecula."

Pathology and primary-site summary stated, "Poorly differentiated squamous cell carcinoma [cancer] transitional cell type of the base of the tongue with metastasis to the jugulodigastric area [neck]."

The patient received 200 rads per day to a total of 6500 rads of cobalt^{60} irradiation.

About two-thirds of the way through the course of this treatment, a new area of cancer involvement manifested itself—the lower right cervical (neck) lymph node area. The upper right had been included in the first field of radiation, and now her doctors planned an additional course. Radiology stated:

> This will be done through a single anterior tangential portal—1500 rads per week for a total of at least 5000 rads with care being taken not to overlap any of the several fields.

The radiation was completed on July 20, 1973, and the patient was requested to return in three weeks. During this period she lost all ability to speak, which, according to the hospital reports, "worried her a great deal" because she could not work unless she could talk.

The patient progressed fairly well, considering the extensive radiation. As late as October 12, 1973 (two and one-half months following radiation), no new swelling of the neck lymph glands or the lymph glands under the arm were noted.

Between October 12, 1973, and November 7, 1973, however, further exams yielded more bad news. In a letter dated November 7, 1973, the Radiology Department of Massachusetts General Hospital advised this patient:

> The lump in your right axilla turns out to be of the same nature as were the glands in the left side of your neck. Therefore, I think you have something further done about this. I would like to give you some X-ray treatment to the place from which the gland was removed. For this you have an appointment with us on Wednesday, November 14, at 10:30 A.M. We will want to see you for treatment three days a week for about three weeks. I have in mind a course of drug treatment which I should like to have instituted so as to increase the security of control of your trouble.

At this point this forty-six-year-old widow decided she had had all the orthodox cure she could handle. One vocal chord was paralyzed, she had lost her voice, her diaphragm was paralyzed, she had had two surgeries on her neck, most of her thyroid was gone, her skin had been burned from the radiation, and her salivary glands had ceased to function—and still do not function. To this day she must carry an atomizer of water in her purse, and, must use it every few minutes to moisten the inside of her mouth.

She declined Harvard Medical School's offer and turned instead to Laetrile, in the hope of controlling the cancerous axillary lymph nodes.

In 1974 she went to a medical doctor in the Southeast for Laetrile treatment, and in September of 1975 came to the Richardson Clinic to continue maintenance therapy.

Our last contact with this patient was on January 5, 1977—two years and two months after she turned down additional radiation to the site of newly developing cancer under her right arm. (The only treatment this area has received is metabolic therapy.) At that time she reported she was in good health, that her voice had returned, and that her cancer apparently had been brought under control.

P117J: Cancer of the Vocal Cords

This man went to Kaiser Hospital in Santa Clara, California, in August of 1971 because of persistent hoarseness and difficulty in speaking.

The vocal cords were biopsied and the pathology report dated August 13, 1971, reads as follows:

> *Gross:*
> The three specimens are imbedded in the order in which they have been identified.
> *Micro + Diagnosis:*
> (1) No demonstrable epithelial atypism right posterior commissure of vocal chords.
> (2) Squamous carcinoma [cancer], right middle commissure of vocal chord.
> (3) Squamous carcinoma, right anterior commissure of vocal chord.

Biopsy is considered one hundred per cent accurate if positive.[1]

Despite the recommendations of the staff, however, this gentleman accepted no surgery, no radiation, and no chemotherapy whatsoever.

He began metabolic therapy August 18, 1971. Within about eight weeks following metabolic therapy his voice returned to normal.

He has had intermittent laryngitis. He does a great deal of talking in connection with his work. The repeated laryngoscopic examinations of the vocal cords

---

[1]*Clinical Oncology for Medical Students and Physicians, op. cit.,* p. 244.

through the years, however, have never revealed a return of the tumor.

This patient's tumor regressed and has not returned. Five and one-half years have passed since the initial diagnosis. The *only* treatment he has received is metabolic therapy.

C147DR: Cancer of the Right Tonsil, Metastatic to the Right Neck

This seventy-six-year-old man went to his local doctor in March, 1974, for an ear examination following a two to three-year history of difficulty in hearing. Examination also revealed an enlarged right tonsil and an enlarged lymph node in the right neck.

On March 4, 1974, this man was admitted to St. Joseph's Hospital, Eureka, California, where his right tonsil was removed. Pathology diagnosis of the frozen section was "lymphocytic lymphosarcoma, well-differentiated." The description of the surgery reads in part as follows:

> It was felt that an excision biopsy would be more likely to reveal the nature of tonsillar enlargement. Therefore, a right tonsillectomy was performed. . . . During the process of hemostasis, a frozen section was performed on the removed tonsil. The pathologist's diagnosis was moderately well to well-differentiated lymphoma. Therefore, the procedure was terminated as the enlarged lymph node must be presumed to be the same pathological entity.

The local physician planned to refer him to another doctor for a complete lymphoma work-up. The finding of positive nodes is a poor prognostic sign. Cure rates (with orthodox treatment) are as low as five per cent.[1]

On April 19, 1974, the local doctor's secretary wrote Mr. C. a note which read in part:

---

[1]*Clinical Oncology for Medical Students and Physicians, op. cit.*, p. 253.

> It is very important that you see a doctor about your cancer. Dr. [name omitted] has been very concerned about your getting help.

The local doctor was advised that the patient wanted to go to the Richardson Clinic, and his records were forwarded.

The patient completed his initial course of metabolic therapy and returned home.

Mr. C. wrote to the Richardson Clinic in April, 1976—two years after his surgery and the diagnostic impression of metastatic cancer of the neck. He states he is still taking the recommended vitamins and following the vegetarian diet, that his health is good for a seventy-six-year-old man, and that his cancer appears to be controlled.

He has had not any radiation or chemotherapy, nor has he had any further surgery.

L128WX: Basal Cell Carcinoma of the Nose

This woman was seventy-four years old at the time of the first biopsy of the side of her nose on August 12, 1971. The diagnosis was basal cell carcinoma.

In a letter dated August 24, 1971, the referring physician stated:

> Patient has basal cell carcinoma of the face involving the left nasal labial area with extension onto the left nasal ala. The lesion is fairly deeply infiltrating, but does not appear to involve the mucous membrane beneath.
>
> Because of the involvement of the ala of the nose, I do not feel that radiation would be the treatment of choice. The deformity following radiation would be quite severe and I think that a better cosmetic result could be obtained with surgical excision. The closure may necessitate a small nasal labial flap.

The patient, who is a nurse, decided in view of her experience to turn down the idea of surgery. She stated she was warned that her face would be gradually eaten away if she did not have surgery.

This lady decided to go on a no-meat diet, yeast, vitamin C, and approximately thirty apricot kernels per day, the latter in divided doses. She stayed on this regimen self-prescribed from September, 1971, until August, 1974.

She began metabolic therapy with the Richardson Clinic in August, 1974. At that time the cancer area at the side of her nose was about the size of a quarter, which, according to patient, was somewhat smaller than it had been two years previously.

A biopsy, December 10, 1974, was returned with a diagnosis of basal cell carcinoma.

The patient continued on the diet, the Laetrile, and vitamin regimen. By November 11, 1975, the area of previous cancerous erosion had almost completely disappeared, and only a smooth scar area remained, with a very small red area visible.

The seventy-four-year-old patient works a full day as a nurse, caring for an eighty-six-year-old invalid. In a letter to the clinic in November, 1975, the patient concluded:

> I feel that the treatment has brought this dread disease under control and has the added benefit of impriving my general health. I I think that had I come earlier in the history of this tumor (had I known of Doctor Richardson) it might have disappeared completely under this treatment. I am grateful to have this available to me, and wish that others suffering greatly with cancer treatment could know of these benefits.

B113M: Cancer of the Nose, Cheek, Throat, and Brain

This woman had a tumor removed from her nostril in 1962.

The patient states that the same area began to cause her discomfort within two months following the 1962 surgery, and she was then given cortisone and radiation therapy.

In 1968 she was seen by a plastic surgeon in Oklahoma City, Oklahoma, who removed a second tumor and part of her nose. Within three months the patient was again having pain at the site of the previous surgeries and received more radiation therapy. The radiation therapy did not control the patient's pain.

In October, 1970, she was referred to Stanford Medical Center in Palo Alto, California, and received 6,000 rads of radiation from the linear accelator. She was told at the time that she would be unable to receive any more radiation at that site. The radiation provided the patient relief from pain until 1973.

During the interval from 1970 to 1973, the patient continued to have routine check-ups and X-rays of the nose area every six months. Despite the return of pain in 1973, she was advised there was "nothing wrong." When the skin broke adjacent to the surgical site and began to drain, further tests were taken and the patient was advised that the cancer had returned.

The patient went to Stanford Medical Center in May, 1974, and had the remainder of her nose and part of the cheek bone amputated. Four months later in September, 1974, the pain had again returned, and the patient called Stanford Medical Center and asked if it were possible to have more radiation to control the discomfort. She was advised she had had all they could give her. She was also advised that she might return and have the other cheek bone removed.

At this point in time Mrs. B. looked into the possible use of metabolic therapy, including the use of Laetrile, at the suggestion of a member of her family. She began metabolic therapy on October 7, 1974. She was seventy-five years old at the time.

In a letter to the Richardson Clinic dated March 4, 1976, (one and one-half years later) the patient describes her response to the treatment in this way.

> I started taking it [Laetrile] and had four shots [one each day for four days] in the vein and immediately started getting relief. . . . I have had one shot a week in the muscle, and two pills a day and have had complete relief.

Before taking Laetril, I was having soreness in my mouth and in my throat; also the cancer had spread up to my brain. This was confirmed by the doctors at Stanford when I had my nose removed.

I feel that Laetril has not killed the cancer but is controlling it.

I saw Dr. G, my medical doctor, six months ago and he checked my nose and said. "Mrs. B., whatever you are doing, continue it."

CENTRAL NERVOUS SYSTEM

Case Histories Include Cancer of the Brain

Complete surgical removal of gliomas (brain cancer) is usually not possible.[1] *Four out of every five patients with cancer of the brain* who do not use Laetrile *but choose surgery and radiation instead will be dead within two years.*[2] *The following Laetrile case histories should be read with these facts in mind.*

C165GX: Brain Tumor: Astrocytoma, Grade II

This woman was thirty-two years old when her symptoms began. She had a six-month history of headaches prior to being hospitalized on May 7, 1975. She had also had several episodes of vomiting.

The admission examination stated in part:

> Examination demonstrated bilateral papilledema [swelling at the back of both eyes]. A cerebral angiography [X-rays showing blood vessels in the brain] demonstrated an avascular mass [a tumor] in the left temporal parietal region [above the ear].

---

[1]*Clinical Oncology for Medical Students and Physicians, op. cit.,* p. 262.
[2]*Ibid,* p. 270.

The dangers of brain surgery were explained to the patient and to her parents. They decided to proceed.

The surgery report dated May 10, 1975, stated in part:

> The tumor measured approximately 8 cm. [about 3 inches] in its greatest dimension. . . . While waiting for the frozen section report an attempt was made to circumvent the tumor . . . from the surrounding normal appearing brain tissue. . . . It soon became evident that this tumor had no real demarcation from the brain tissue from which it arose. . . .
>
> Once it became clear that this tumor arose from the brain itself, no further attempt was made to circumvent this tumor mass. . . . Removal of the tumor by suctioning was continued until "normal appearing" white matter was encountered.

The operation was described as a "Left temporal parietal craniotomy with *incomplete* excision of astrocytoma, low grade."

Pathology diagnosis was "Fibrillary Astrocytoma with Microcyst Formation (Grade II)."

Surgery was followed by twenty-seven radiation treatments, which the patient tolerated fairly well. These were begun on May 21, 1975.

According to Joseph Mc Donald, M.D., and Lowell Lapham, M.D., "Most glioblastoma [astrocytoma] patients recur and die within the first year."[1]

In this woman's case, she was having recurrence of symptoms two months following surgery and radiation. The left side of her face had become swollen, and headaches and nausea had returned.

No attempt was made at this point to determine whether the tumor was recurring or radionecrosis was causing the problem.

---

[1]*Clinical Oncology for Medical Students and Physicians, op. cit.*, p. 270.

On July 3, 1975, this patient was brought to the Richardson Clinic, after she had been advised by the surgeon that nothing more could be done.

Blood studies were essentially normal. Minerals were balanced following hair analysis. The patient received 9 gms. of Laetrile I.V. for twenty days and then gradually decreased I.V. dosage supplemented by oral medication on the days she did not receive I.V. The headaches were gradually reduced in severity, and in five months they were completely gone.

Bio-assays since starting metabolic therapy have been: (1) 7-3-75, 19.0, (2) 7-25-75, 16.7, (3) 8-22-75, 14.9, (4) 919-75, 14.5, (5) 1-26-76, 14.6, (6) 6-9-76, 15.7[1]

This woman is alive and well nearly two years following the incomplete removal of a brain tumor.

The patient's father stated in a letter to Dr. Richardson dated January 2, 1977:

> At the end of the treatment our doctor [the surgeon] told me that she [the patient] should still try to enjoy herself which she could, for she might be able to live six months, a year or, at most, two years.
>
> This meant that orthodox medicine could do no more for her. At the end of our rope we took our daughter to your clinic on July 3, 1975. In October, 1975, she was able to return to work full time and has since been leading a normal life.
>
> My daughter and I are shocked and indignant to learn that Big Brother is prosecuting you for saving lives. We vow that if necessary we'll fight along side you for our right to live.

S135G: Cancer of the Brain

Mr. S. was found to have cancer of the brain in December, 1970. He wanted to go on metabolic therapy including Laetrile, but the Richardson Clinic recommended to him that he first have the surgery his

---

[1]See appendix for normals.

doctor had suggested, and then come to the clinic.

Surgery was performed January 7, 1971. The patient was told that they could not get all the cancer and, even with some radiation therapy, he could not possibly live more than six months.

The patient came to the Richardson Clinic early in 1971 and has continued faithfully on the metabolic therapy program.

Four years later in July, 1975, the Sacramento, California, Sutter Hospital acquired a new scanner. The patient had a brain scan at the time and was told he did not have a trace of cancer.

He continues to be in good health and leads a normal, active life.

CANCER OF THE BONE

Patients with osteogenic sarcoma (bone cancer) who do not use Laetrile *but choose surgery and/or radiation instead usually die within 12 to 18 months following diagnosis.*[1] *The following case histories should be read with this fact in mind.*

H150S: Osteosarcoma Right Humerus (Cancer of the Right Upper Arm Bone) with Metastasis

This little boy was six years old when his symptoms first began. He had been a normal, active youngster and then over a short period of time became listless and complained of pain in his thighs and arm. The parents went to the child's pediatrician in July, 1973, and were referred to a bone specialist. The orthopedist felt there was nothing to be concerned about and, according to the parents, advised them to go ahead with a planned vacation. Apparently no diagnostic X-rays were taken.

The child became so weak during the vacation that he had to see Disneyland from a wheelchair. Upon returning to their northern Nevada home, the parents sought a physical therapist because the boy could no longer stand straight or run.

In October, 1973, a new symptom presented itself. Little Shane, who was right-handed, began trying to use his left hand. The mother describes watching

[1]*Textbook of Radiotherapy*, Second Edition, by Gilbert H. Fletcher, M.D. (Lea and Febiger, Philadelphia, 1973), p. 556.

him at dinner one night and asking him why he was eating left-handed. His response was to look at her with a helpless, puzzled expression which indicated he just did not know how to explain his problem. He could do no more than shrug his shoulders, and then, using his left hand, he raised his right arm and rested it on the table.

His mother asked him to stand up and show her how high he could raise his right arm. Her heart sank. He could raise it only from the elbow, not from the shoulder. In the light of the earlier reassurance from an orthopedic doctor that nothing was wrong, she stated that she was "terribly confused."

On November 6, 1973, the parents again sought the help of a physical therapist and on the same day asked the doctor to look at Shane again. The area of the humerus [right upper arm bone] was warm to the touch, and the doctor sent the child for X-rays. The X-ray findings did not indicate a break but rather bone disease, so the child was admitted to the hospital the same evening for a complete check-up.

The conclusion of the physicians, based on the X-rays, and bone marrow biopsy, was osteosarcoma of the right humerus and also of the third lumbar vertebra (spine). The parents were advised that the child's chances were "grim."

The pathology report of the bone marrow biopsy from Mercy Hospital, Sacramento, California, dated November 9, 1973, stated:

> The specimen consisted of approximately 20 irregularly-shaped masses of soft grey neoplastic tissue, the largest measuring 20 x 9 x 5 mm. Included were a few very small spicules of bone. . . .
>
> Microscopically, the masses consisted almost entirely of fairly large round and spindle-shaped neoplastic cells. The tumor cells contained pleomorphic moderately hyperchromatic nuclei. Many of the cells were arranged in broad sheets interspersed with osteoid tissue, showing partial ossification. There were large numbers of mitotic

figures. The tumor cells were infiltrated between bony spicules. Some portions of the tumor appeared cartilaginous, but the multiple foci of osteoid tissue indicated that the lesion was an osteosarcoma. The lesion did not show the giant cell formation and focal calcification found in chondroblastomas.

Diagnosis:

Osteosarcoma (osteogenic sarcoma) [cancer] in tissue from the right humerus.

Comment:

These slides were reviewed by my associate [name omitted] who concurs with the diagnosis.

The hospital summary of November 11, 1973, stated in part:

> It would appear that this unfortunate child has already distant metastases from his primary tumor. In all likelihood he will develop evidence of metastases elsewhere in the very near future . . . pulmonary metastases are so common with metastatic osteogenic sarcoma. Unfortunately the patient is not a candidate for curative therapy and the primary question is how best to palliate this child to maintain him in a functional painfree state for as long as possible.

Radiation was decided upon as the treatment of choice. The radiologist pointed out, however, that, because the child had metastasis to the third lumbar vertebra (cancer of the spinal column bone) *in addition* to his cancer of the right upper arm bone, there would be no point in subjecting him to a high dose of radiation (5,000 to 8,000+ rads per site) to render the cancer "quiescent" prior to amputation. The child was going to die from the metastasis regardless of what was done to the arm. The radiologist planned 2,500 rads to the arm and 2,000 rads to the spine to "palliate" (not cure) the cancer. In his recommendation the radiologist stated, "Although this is not a lesion which responds well to radiation therapy, I believe irradiation of the areas of known disease should cause some degree of restraint of tumor growth [and] . . . should lengthen the patient's pain free period."

The parents were told in November, 1973, the child had six to nine months to live. The lesions were too extensive for long-term control.

The child's mother stated that news of their tragedy spread quickly, and many people offered help. She was told about the success cancer patients were having in Mexico at Laetrile clinics. Later, she found out about the Richardson Clinic, which was closer to her home.

Little Shane began metabolic therapy including Laetrile on November 29, 1973. His alkaline phosphatase at the beginning of treatment was an incredible 1,250 mu/ml, (lab normals, 30-85 mu/ml). Repeat analysis verified the original finding. Hemoglobin, hematocrit and segs were all slightly low. Lymphs were 63%, (lab normals, 20-40%).

Within a month after beginning metabolic therapy, he was able to use his arm a little and was no longer carrying it in a sling. The pain gradually decreased, and his energy returned. Alkaline phosphatase had dropped to 195 mu/ml by March 21, 1974.

The patient's mother wrote a letter to the Richardson Clinic in May, 1976, two and one-half years after being told her child's chances were "grim". The letter reads in part as follows:

> Now he will even try to throw a ball with it [the right arm]. He has gained weight and seems to flourish and grow as a normal child.
>
> I feel fantastic about what happened.
>
> We took him to see . . . [a local physician] at the doctor's request in April, 1974. He X-rayed Shane and found improvement. He wouldn't give vitamin therapy any credit for this but made some comment about not stopping what I was doing.

The patient's mother found it necessary temporarily to discontinue the vitamins in May, 1976, because of financial problems, but she tried to have her child adhere to the diet as much as possible. It is not an easy task to keep an active nine-year-old on a diet which, among other things, is free of all sources of refined sugar.

The mother's letter concluded, "Due to my religious beliefs, I could take death but not the pain—not for a little child. I could see no reason for a six-year-old to have to suffer before death." Her love for her child and her unwillingness to see him suffer brought her to Laetrile. It matters little to the mother whether her local doctor is annoyed with her not using "orthodox" therapy.

This child returned to the Richardson clinic for a check-up in January, 1977. He was sent to Albany Hospital, Albany, California, for X-rays. The arm looked so good the radiologist could not believe the child ever had osteosarcoma. He was not aware that the bone marrow biopsy diagnosis had been verified by two pathologists. He was also unaware that the child had not had a full course of X-ray therapy. The X-ray report dated January 24, 1977, stated in part:

> *Right Humerus:*
> Films of the right humerus show marked shortening of this bone. There is angular deformity noted in one view, suggestive of old spontaneous fracture. Several sharply defined cystic areas in the shaft. Epiphysis sclerotic and the epiphyseal line is probably open. There is an irregular area of bone destruction simulating a marginal erosion at the lateral aspect of the epiphyseal line. No subperiosteal new bone and no soft tissue mass.
> *Conclusion:*
> Findings as above. History of previous osteogenic sarcoma with X-ray therapy. Clinical course and findings atypical and I would wonder if this was not either an eosinphilic granuloma or a Ewing's sarcoma.

Osteogenic sarcoma is considered radio resistant. As stated previously, radiation in high doses (5,000 to 8,000+ rads) is used, however, to render the cancer "quiescent" prior to surgical removal by amputation.[1] Inoperable osteogenic sarcoma has a survival rate of practically zero.

This child is alive and well more than three years following the initial diagnosis. Until Laetrile is openly accepted—thereby coming under insurance coverage and tax deductibility, thus easing the financial burden—the lives of children like Shane will be sacrificed needlessly.

Shane's photograph and reproductions of his 1973 and 1977 X-rays appear elsewhere in this book.

R160PA: Metastatic Cancer of the Bone, Previous Cancer of the Prostate

Mr. A. had his prostate removed in 1966. The diagnosis was adenocarcenoma, according to Kaiser Hospital in Walnut Creek, California.

In 1974, this patient had bone scans. A hospital report dated January 7, 1976, stated in part:

> At that time the patient was noted to have increased pain, and a bone scan showed multiple abnormal sites of concentration in the rib cage and sternum and vertebral column as well as the posterior pelvis. The medial portion of the right knee was also quite warm. X-rays showed a diffuse sclerosis of the dorsal vertebrae, suspicious of osteoblastic metastasis [cancer] since the sclerosis was not present on films taken a year earlier. Accordingly, 9/24/74, he was started on Stilbesterol, one mgm. daily with good relief of his pain.
>
> His most recent examination was October 3, 1975, at which time he seemed to have no additional symptoms but continued to have some pain, probably related to his pre-existing osteoarthritic problem, particularly of the knee.

The patient states that after the diagnosis of cancer of the bone he "went into a deep depression." He

---

[1]*Clinical Oncology for Medical Students and Physicians, op. cit.,* pp. 293, 294.

experienced loss of appetite, loss of equilibrium, insomnia, lack of bladder control and "all over weakness."

Some of these symptoms are associated with patients using Stilbesterol. One of the drug companies producing Stilbesterol lists among the "side effects" of taking Stilbesterol the following: (1) anxiety, (2) vertigo (in which the subject has difficulty maintaining equilibrium), (3) insomnia, and (4) lassitude (a feeling of "all over weakness," to use the patient's expression).

The seventy-eight-year-old man stated that, after encouragement from several people who had benefited from vitamin therapy, he decided to go to the Richardson Clinic. Metabolic therapy including Laetrile was begun December 30, 1975.

The patient indicated that 1976, the first year on metabolic therapy, was a much better year than 1975. He described the results as "spectacular" both mentally and physically. He experienced a decided gain in energy and stated he has had no further depression, pain, or stomach distress.

Stilbesterol is at best only a temporary control for the symptoms of bone cancer,[1] and its use carries with it the risk of thrombo-embolus[2] (a floating blood clot) formation, which is particularly risky among older people, whose blood vessels may already be partly plugged. The patient may die of a heart attack or stroke *because* of his use of female hormones to palliate (not cure) his bone cancer. He would then become a heart attack or stroke statistic and not appear on the record as having died from cancer.

This patient's symptom-free year on metabolic therapy including Laetrile does not involve this kind of risk.

---

[1]*Clinical Oncology for Medical Students and Physicians, op. cit.*, p. 206.

[2]*Ibid.*, p. 206.

CANCER OF THE ENDOCRINE GLANDS

Case Histories Include Cancer of the Thyroid

Cancer of the thyroid is very slow growing and, therefore, it is not unusual to find cases involving five-year survival following orthodox therapy. Surgical removal of the thyroid, however, can result in nerve paralysis.[1] *Leukemia has been shown to be related to the previous use of radioactive iodine to treat cancer of the thyroid.*[2] *The following case history should be read with these facts in mind.*

A156JC: Cancer of the Thyroid

Mrs. A. noticed a lump on her neck in March, 1973. The lump was removed and, because of the diagnosis of cancer, further surgery was performed two days later. Following surgery, the radioactive thyroid scan was negative.

Despite assurance from her doctor that all was well, the patient herself described being constantly tired and feeling a lump in her throat during the summer of 1973.

September, 1973, a second radioactive thyroid scan was done, and this time it was positive, indicating the presence of cancer. Therefore, a radical thyroid

---

[1]*Clinical Oncology for Medical Students and Physicians, op. cit.*, p. 320.
[2]*Ibid.*, p. 321.

gland removal, including removal of muscle and lymph nodes, was performed. This was done in October of 1973. It was followed by an "Atomic Cocktail," (presumably, a drink of radio-active iodine) which, she stated, was supposed to "wipe out the rest of the cancer."

What happened next is described in the patient's own words:

> I recovered slowly through the winter of 1973. . . . Then in July, 1974, my health really went down hill. I lost about thirty pounds. I had yellow dark skin[1] and dark around my eyes. I was constantly tired. I slept a great deal and felt sleepy the rest of the time. It was around this time I first heard of Laetrile. I felt the treatments I had been receiving were ineffective, and so I chose to come to the Richardson Clinic.
>
> Dr. Richardson did not make any promises to me, but within *ten* days of beginning nutritional therapy and Laetrile, I noted considerable improvement. My eyes and skin returned to their normal color. I stopped losing weight, the terrible tired feeling left, as did the pain. . . .
>
> Friends and relatives who have watched my progress are amazed at how well I look. . . . We've had a number of cases of cancer in my family on both sides. I am the only one who has taken Laetrile and I am the only one who has survived.

---

[1]Yellowing of the skin is a very ominous sign—indicating liver involvement.

CANCER OF THE LYMPH SYSTEM

Case Histories Include Hodgkin's Disease

Patients with Hodgkin's Disease who do not use Laetrile *but choose orthodox therapy instead have a better statistical chance of long-term survival than those with most forms of cancer. This is because, as a rule, it does not progress rapidly. One person in five, however, will die as a result of the side-effects of radiation or chemotherapy.*[1] *(Typical causes of death are pneumonia, blood poisoning, tuberculosis, or fungus infections.) It is important to note also that Hodgkin's Disease patients who accept radiation and chemotherapy develop cancer at secondary sites at a rate twenty-nine times greater than those who accept no treatment at all.*[2] *The use of Laetrile and metabolic therapy does not include such risks. These facts should be kept in mind when reading the following case histories.*

J154LT: Nodular Sclerosing Hodgkin's Disease, Stage IV-B

Just prior to her sixteenth birthday the once active, alert teenage girl was diagnosed as having Hodgkin's Disease.

---

[1]Ultmann, *et al.:* "The Clinical Picture of Hodgkin's Disease," *Cancer Research,* 26:1047, 1966.
[2]Arseneau, *et al.:* "Recently Recognized Complications of Cancer Chemotherapy" *Annals of the New York Academy of Sciences,* Vol. 230, *op. cit.,* pp. 483, 484.

In March, 1974, a lymph node in her neck was biopsied at a hospital near her Coeur D'Alene, Idaho, home. The results of that biopsy began a nightmare for this young lady.

Her spleen was removed in April, 1974, and the girl's parents were advised that she would have to have approximately one month of daily cobalt treatments as soon as she recovered from the surgery. These were administered from mid-April to mid-May, 1974. Later, the parents and Miss J. were told she would have to have chemotherapy consisting of nitrogen mustard[1] plus Matulane and Prednisone. This was administered from late-August through late-September, 1974.

Blood platelet count during the period of chemotherapy ranged from 815,000 to 165,000 (lab normals, 140-440 mil.). Her white blood count varied from 17,300 (which coincided with a lung X-ray change indicating probable inflammation on September 9, 1974) down to 5,500 on September 2, 1974 (lab normals, 4-10,000 min).

The Idaho hospital sent ten of this patient's pathology slides to Stanford University Medical Center in Los Altos, California, on July 5, 1974, with a request that the university evaluate them. The Idaho hospital identified her as having "Hodgkin's Disease involving the mediastinum, spleen, and intra abdominal lymph nodes with subsequent development of sixth nerve palsy . . . and a recent left posterior iliac crest needle biopsy contains a disturbing lesion." Stanford's diagnosis based on the slides was:

1. *left cervical (neck) mass, biopsy—consistent with Hodgkin's disease, nodular sclerosing type.*
2. *Spleen, splenectomy—nodular sclerosing Hodgkin's disease.*

---

[1]It should be noted that it is against the Geneva Convention to use nitrogen mustard against an enemy in war.

3. Bone marrow, iliac crest, needle biopsy—focal involvement by Hodgkin's disease.[1]

The technicality of all these data does not tell us what this sixteen-year-old girl was going through as a result of her diagnosis and the best efforts of her doctors to save her life.

The following description of what Miss J. went through is taken from a letter her father wrote to his company's insurance carrier. First he describes her orthodox treatment as he saw it:

> Radiation treatments were to start as soon as she had recovered from her splenectomy. During this time, the size of the swelling on her neck increased four to five times, as if it were angry from being disturbed.
>
> Radiation therapy, which did reduce the swelling, brought on nausea and loss of appetite. By the time the twenty-six treatments were complete she weighed 105 pounds.
>
> Our daughter had chills and fever and she was burned on her neck and under her arms. Many nights her bed and nightgown were sopping wet and had to be changed three or four times. Sometimes within a period of twenty minutes the sweats would change to chills so bad her teeth would chatter.
>
> My wife and I would attempt to relieve the chilling by heating blankets in the dryer and many nights the blankets were changed every five or ten minutes for a period of an hour. The doctor recommended aspirin to relieve her fevers.
>
> During this same time our daughter would have leg aches so bad she would sit doubled up with tears in her eyes. The doctor stated the leg aches were from the fevers and to take aspirin for relief.
>
> Following the radiation during a rest period from treatment she began to see double when she

---

[1]In Hodgkin's Disease, Stage IV means the disease has extended to the bone marrow, lung, pleura, skin, gastrointestinal tract, liver or other non-lymph tissue. The designation "B" means the patient has fever, night sweats, and/or itching.

looked straight ahead and she lost the ability to look to the left out of her left eye. The doctor was called for an eye exam and our daughter was told her sight would never return to normal. She went to a neurologist who ran many tests including a brain wave and spinal tap. No specific cause of the eye problem was suggested to us.

During this time she continued to grow weaker and had no appetite whatsoever despite the fact that the radiation treatments were finished. She continued to have chills and fever, and leg aches. She lost hair no the back of her head.

Because her bone marrow tests were positive she was scheduled for chemotherapy.

One of the drugs created an acute ugly acne condition on her face. We were told this usually happened.

For thirty minutes before the nitrogen mustard injections and for fifteen minutes afterward her head was packed in ice to reduce the chance of hair loss. Five minutes prior to the injection a small rubber tube was fixed tightly around her head to reduce the blood circulation.

The injections also killed good blood cells and caused the walls of the veins to deteriorate which made it very difficult to obtain the required daily blood samples. The blood vessels in our daughter's arm were turning brown. The doctor advised us they were dead, but not to worry; there were plenty of veins to take care of the circulation.

During the "rest period" of the first chemotherapy cycle (between the 14th and 28th day) she began to develop a dry hacking cough. X-rays showed cloudy areas in the lungs and the doctor could not determine whether they were caused from cobalt or cancer without doing exploratory surgery, which we would not allow. Lee had already suffered so much.

The hacking cough continued to worsen during and after completion of the second chemotherapy cycle. By the time we made the decision to go to the Richardson Clinic, the cough was

> constant except for occasional no coughing periods of no longer than three minutes.
>
> By the end of the second chemotherapy cycle Lee had fevers of 104° and more chills and severe leg cramps. She was taking aspirin every four hours day and night. She was very weak, had no appetite and would only drink one glass of water all day.
>
> From the beginning of the fall term of school in late August, 1974, until November 4, 1974, she was able to attend school only three days.
>
> She was so weak she was seldom up more than four hours a day. She went only to the doctor's office and then back home to her bedroom to lie down.
>
> Her mother and I felt our daughter's life was being poisoned away by the toxicity of the chemicals and the burning of the radiation.

This is the background against which the decision to seek metabolic therapy was made. This teenager came to the Richardson Clinic and began treatment October 2, 1974. She was practically carried into the clinic by her parents because she was so weak she could hardly walk.

Miss J's father continues to explain to the insurance carrier, in a letter dated April 16, 1975, what happened following the change in treatment modalities:

> Six days after beginning metabolic therapy the cough was gone, and only returned temporarily during a winter cold.
>
> A calcium shot was given her which immediately relieved her leg aches.
>
> Upon returning home after the initial twenty injections, Lee began attending school. By this time she no longer had the high fevers, chills, leg aches, or continuous coughs. Her appetite increased.
>
> In January, 1975, she returned to Albany, California, for a check-up. She had gained eleven pounds, still had a good appetite, and still no fever, chills, etc.
>
> During the winter semester she only missed

twelve and one-half days of school, five of which she was home with Herpes, three days she went to the doctor's office in California, two days she had the flu, and two days she had an ear infection.

At this writing she continues to gain strength, is generally feeling well, goes out with her boyfriend, and has signed up for a night class which meets for three hours twice a week.

The letter was written in the hope that the insurance company would be willing to pay for the metabolic therapy which was costing about half as much as the previous cobalt and chemotherapy treatments. (The surgeries and diagnostic studies were not included in that financial summary. If they had been, the cost difference would have been even greater.) Sadly, the insurance company would have gladly paid for additional chemotherapy at twice the price, but it would not pay one cent for metabolic therapy.

Miss J. now works part time and continues her schooling. It has been more than two years since she abandoned orthodox therapy in favor of metabolic therapy, and she continues to lead a symptom-free and active life of a normal healthy teenager.

K112MJ: Hodgkin's Disease, Stage II-B

This twenty-six-year-old woman was pregnant at the time she first began to feel that there was a lump in the back of her throat.

Diagnostic X-rays were postponed until after delivery in mid-October, 1975. X-rays and a biopsy of the largest lymph node on the patient's neck confirmed the diagnosis of Hodgkin's Disease, probable clinical Stage II-B.[1]

Reports from the University Hospital, University of Washington, Seattle, Washington, read in part as follows:

---

[1]In Hodgkin's Disease, Stage II means the disease involves more than two areas but is confined to one side of the diaphragm only. The designation "B" means the patient has fever, night sweats, and/or itching.

Chest X-rays, November 4, 1975
Impression: Large anterior mediastinal and retrosternal lymph nodes compatible with lymphoma.
Pathology Report, November 6, 1975
Specimen: Supraclavicular node biopsy
Diagnosis: Hodgkin's disease, nodular sclerosing type (cellular phase).
Liver Scan, November 10, 1975
Impression: Normal liver and spleen scan. Bone Marrow Report, November 10, 1975
Impression: No evidence of involvement of the bone marrow.
Lymphangiogram, November 12, 1975
Conclusion: Normal pedal lymphangiogram without evidence of abdominal Hodgkin's disease.

Exploratory surgery to determine the extent of involvement was strongly recommended, but the patient rfeused for rligious reasons.

The patient was considering accepting the recommended radiation and chemotherapy when she heard about metabolic therapy and Laetrile. She first came to the Richardson Clinic on January 8, 1976.

In her words:

> It seemed to make so much sense, and after much prayer we decided to make an appointment with Dr. Richardson. It was a little "scarey" for the first couple of days [because they weren't following their local doctor's recommendations], but our confidence was boosted after several days of sitting in the waiting room talking to the different ones that had really been helped with vitamin therapy. After three weeks of my treatments, I was convinced.

The patient stated that her local doctor is pleased with her apparent improvement, for there has been a reduction in the size of the lymph nodes.

The patient states she still gets tired and tries to take naps, but she is continuing to stay on the diet and vitamins, and her condition is responding favorably as of our last contact.

CANCER OF THE BLOOD AND BLOOD-FORMING SYSTEMS

The Leukemias

Reliable statistics on death rates among chronic leukemia patients are difficult to find. Orthodoxy speaks in terms of a "median survival" of only three years,[1] *and admits that the effects of currently accepted therapy have not been adequately evaluated.*[2]

The use of one of the chemotherapy drugs of choice, Leukeran, carries with it the risk of irreversible damage to the bone marrow. Another chemotherapy drug, Cytoxan, has produced cancer in rats and mice. Some of the reactions Cytoxan has produced in humans include: nausea, vomiting, bleeding and inflammation of the colon, severe bleeding from the bladder, and in males, possible irreversible loss of sperm production.[3] *The use of metabolic therapy does not involve these kinds of risks. These facts should be kept in mind while reading the following case histories.*

---

[1]*Clinical Oncology for Medical Students and Physicians, op. cit.*, p. 371.

[2]*Ibid.*, p. 370.

[3]This information is supplied by the drug manufacturer, each vial or bottle of tablets describing the drug's dosage, use, and dangers. The doctor is free, as a rule, to decide how much information any particular patient will receive.

R106B: Chronic Lymphatic Leukemia

On July 3, 1973, this sixty-two-year-old man went to his local doctor because he had developed a lump on his neck. One week later, this was biopsied, and because of the findings he was referred to a blood and cancer specialist in Sacramento, California. The consulting physician's summary dated August 6, 1973, reads in part:

> I feel confident that he had chronic lymphatic leukemia. As you know, histologically the pathologists are not able to determine on the basis of a biopsy whether it is lymphosarcoma or chronic lymphatic leukemia. In recent years both of these have been grouped together in the so-called lymphoproliferative disease group. I think the final diagnosis depends upon the amount of involvement of abnormal lymphoid tissue.
>
> In this case, I note left axillary and left inguinal adenopathy and also the scar from the biopsy of a node in the right supraclavicular area.
>
> It was my feeling that he also had an enlarged spleen.
>
> We obtained on July 27, 1973, a hemoglobin of 15 gm., with a 47% hematocrit. The white count was 24,000 [lab normals, 5,000-10,000], due to an 84% mature lymphocytosis. The platelet count was 211,000 and the reticulocyte count was 1.4%. The direct Coombs' was negative. Serum uric acid 6.3 mg.%; creatinine 1.1 mg.%.
>
> I obtained a liver-spleen scan, a copy of which is enclosed. As you can see, there was considerable enlargement of the spleen noted.
>
> I obtained a bone marrow biopsy which indicated approximately 60% infiltration of the bone marrow by mature lymphocytes.

The patient was started on Vincristine 2 mg. I.V. weekly, Cytoxan three times a day for one week with recommendation it be cut down to 50 mg. two times a day, and Prednisone 14 mg. morning and evening.

Mr. R. states that a few days after his lump was

diagnosed as chronic lymphatic leukemia a friend approached him and his wife with information about Laetrile. He stated he will be "eternally grateful" for the information. On July 23, 1973, he began metabolic therapy including Laetrile.

In a letter to the Richardson Clinic dated February 20, 1976, he summarized his reaction to the diagnosis and the suggested treatments.

> I took chemotherapy for three days only. I had started metabolic therapy on July 23 and 24 [1973] and then submitted [for the last time] to the chemotherapy on July 27, 1973. Mixed up? Yes. But, then what does one do for cancer treatment when one knows nothing to start with?
>
> It took only a few minutes reading in the *Physician's Desk Reference* on the third day I was on chemotherapy to know what I wanted to do and what I did not want to do. This is what the book had to say aobut my drugs: *"Ovocen (Vincristine):* Mode of action is unknown but under investigation. . . . Extreme care must be used in calculating the dose. . . Overdosing may have a serious or fatal outcome." *Cytoxin:* "Its mechanism of action is not known."
>
> Nor did I want *Prednisone,* about which I read more of the same.
>
> I was not ready to die, not from cancer and certainly not from the poisons they were going to give me, so I wouldn't die from cancer.

The patient states that, prior to his metabolic therapy treatment, although he had worked hard every day, he did not feel that he was in as vigorous good health as he could be.

This sixty-five-year-old gentleman and his wife were interviewed at length in November, 1975, two years and four months following the initiation of metabolic therapy. The patient's eyes sparkled like a young man's, and his skin was clear and tight. He had a handsome grey beard that would have been a photographer's delight. His mannerism was animated.

He stated that, before beginning metabolic therapy

including Laetrile, and adopting a vegetarian diet, his mind was confused and his disposition "not that good." He stated he feels much better now and concluded:

> There is no sacrifice I would not willingly make in the culinary field in order to be in vigorous good health. I cannot understand people who say they cannot live this way. All they are doing is confusing self-indulgence with self-love. If you love yourself you should not find it that hard to use a bit of self-discipline and give up your old ways, including coffee, alcohol and cigarettes so that you can get more joy out of living. That is the Lord's way and His way is the way I'm going to go.

He and his wife of many years turned their grey heads toward one another and smiled tenderly. He took her hand in his and looked up at me and said, "Thanks to Dr. Richardson, I'm a whole man now."

Mr. R. continues to lead an active life three and one-half years following the diagnosis of leukemia. With the exception of three days of chemotherapy he has had no treatment other than metabolic therapy including Laetrile.

H155C: Leukemia

This little girl was twelve years old at the time of her initial diagnosis of leukemia. She was on Methotroxate and Cytoxin chemotherapy for approximately one year.

The parents of the patient were not satisfied with their child's progress because she continued to grow weak. They took her first to Dr. Contreras in Mexico and later to the Richardson Clinic where she began metabolic therapy including Laetrile on January 22, 1975. Her alkaline phosphatase was 134 mu/ml at that time (laboratory normal 30-85 mu/ml). White blood count was low (4,900 cu.mm) due to previous chemotherapy.

Miss C. has continued on her maintenance program

of diet and vitamins. She has returned to school and enjoys horseback riding.

Blood studies, dated April 12, 1976, returned to the Richardson Clinic from the child's home in New Jersey showed the alkaline phosphatase to be 12.00 i.u./1. (lab normals, 10-50). The white blood count was 5,000 (lab normals, 4,800-10,800).

In a letter dated July 20, 1976 (one and one-half years after the patient began metabolic therapy), the following statement was made by the patient's physician in New Jersey:

> At [name omitted] last examination 7/7/76, she was in excellent health. There are no palpable lymph nodes or palpable organs. Her skin was free of bruises.

The patient's mother wrote the Richardson Clinic in February, 1977, and said she continues to be an apparently healthy, active teenager with no trace of her former disease.

K127J: Chronic Lymphocytic Leukemia

This fifty-three-year-old male had a peripheral bone marrow smear on May 9, 1975, at St. John's Hospital in Longview, Washington. The diagnosis was chronic lymphocytic leukemia. Physician's comment at the time was as follows:

> Leukemia at the present time is regarded as in the early stages and well differentiated. If there are no other clinical problems and signs of the disease, it might be appropriate to observe the patient over a period of time obtaining CBC's at three or six month intervals.

The patient decided that, rather than wait until his health began to deteriorate, he would begin metabolic therapy. He started treatment May 29, 1975. The patient noticed he had more energy and was sleeping better within a week.

In a letter dated April 19, 1976, almost a year later, the patient stated he has been careful about following the diet and continuing the maintenance program of Laetrile, other vitamins, and enzymes. His general health has remained good and he remains free of the symptoms associated with Leukemia. His white blood count has gradually gone down from 15,000 to 12,000 (10,000 being the high end of normal).

W130B: Chronic Myelogenous Leukemia

This thirty-nine-year-old woman was found to have a white blood count of 73,000 during a routine physical examination in January, 1973. Subsequent bone marrow studies referred to three different laboratories all confirmed the diagnosis of leukemia.

Further studies at the Virginia Mason Clinic in Seattle, Washington, reconfirmed the diagnosis. She was placed on Myleran and Zylorprim, after having had their possible adverse side effects explained to her.

Mrs. W. continued to follow the recommendations of the Virginia Mason Clinic until July, 1975, at which time she came to the Richardson Clinic for metabolic therapy including Laetrile. Her white blood count has continued to stay within normal limits as of this writing, and the patient stated she feels "so much better" than before beginning metabolic therapy. It is, of course, possible that this is a natural remission and that at some future time her white blood count might again climb. However, the patient has already been spared ten months of palliative treatment with Myleran, an alkylating agent whose possible toxic side effects include: skin hyperpigmentation (changes in skin color), irreversible pulmonary fibrosis (formation of scar tissue in the connective tissue framework of the lungs leaving the patient permanently unable to breathe properly), and renal damage (kidney damage).

A102SM: Chronic Lymphatic Leukemia

This sixty-two-year-old male, Doctor of Chiropractic, first developed symptoms of extreme weakness and night sweats in October, 1972. Prior to that he had had a gradual weight loss of twenty-five pounds.

In December, 1972, he went to his local M.D. Subsequent laboratory exams showed an elevated WBC (white blood count) of 350,000 and a depressed RBC (red blood count) of 4.0 gms. The diagnosis of chronic lymphatic leukemia was made. Chest X-rays were negative for mediastinal node and lung involvement. By January 16, 1973, his WBC had risen to 710,000, seventy-one times normal.

His initial contact with the Richardson Clinic was February 1, 1973. The patient's chief complaint was extreme fatigue. He was jaundiced and his liver and spleen were enlarged. The patient began metabolic therapy on his first visit.

During the course of the next six months, his strength increased and he was able to resume most of his chiropractic duties. The jaundice gradually decreased and the liver and spleen could no longer be felt. The liver was still moderately tender in July, 1973, however.

In addition to the metabolic therapy regimen, the patient was on Predneslone every other day as a control for his hemolytic (destruction of red blood cells) tendency. The patient's WBC continued to be elevated, around 200,000 per cu. mm., but he manifested none of the other symptoms usually associated with chronic lymphatic leukemia, which are: enlarged liver and spleen, extreme weakness, jaundice, and hemorrhage.

In February, 1974, this patient decided to discontinue his Laetrile therapy. By May 14, 1974, his WBC had risen to 815,000 per cu.mm. (eighty-one times normal) and his hemoglobin (RBC) had dropped to 5.0 gm. His spleen and liver could be felt again. He became jaundiced and was bothered by ankle edema.

He returned to his metabolic therapy program, and his June 14, 1974, hemotology (blood study) report revealed WBC 595,000 per cu.mm. and hemoglobin 8.9 gm.

This patient continues to have a WBC which is considerably above normal (lab high normal, 10,000), averaging around 200,000. As of this writing, however, the patient—who, three years ago, was too weak to work—is able to carry on his daily routine as if he did not have leukemia, provided he stays on his diet and medication.

F121G: Chronic Lymphatic Leukemia, Coronary Artery Disease, and Bronchitis

Mr. F. first began to have difficulty with enlarged axillary (under arm) lymph nodes in January, 1974. According to the patient, his local doctor was not particularly concerned despite repeated complaints.

In October of 1974, Mr. F. sought another physician's opinion and was subsequently admitted to a hospital in Livermore, California, for diagnostic studies. These confirmed the diagnoses of leukemia.

The patient states the diagnosis made him quite depressed because he had watched his daughter die slowly from cancer. The memories of her last days and the morphine injections made him determined not to have any radiation or chemotherapy.

About this time, another daughter of his had been reading about Laetrile and metabolic therapy and suggested that her father try it.

The patient began metabolic therapy in November of 1974. The lymph nodes gradually decreased in size. Mr. F. stated that he began to feel better and no longer had pain shortly after beginning treatment. He gained weight and stated that, in his opinion, even the heart pain was less of a problem.[1]

Following the initial course of therapy, he returned to his local doctor for a routine check-up. Upon the doctor's advice, he was X-rayed again, and the X-

---

[1]This may have been due to the simultaneous use of vitamin B_{15} (Pangamic Acid). An extensive review of the findings of medical researchers as to the actions of this vitamin is available in the anthology titled, *Vitamin B_{15} (Pangamic Acid) Properties, Functions and Use,* authored by more than thirty scientists, 205 pp. (Available from American Media.)

rays were negative for regional lymphadenopathy (enlarged lymph nodes) indicating the cancer was under control.

The patient stated he intends to remain on a maintenance dose of B_{17} because, in his opinion, it not only has extended his life but has saved him from the tortures of orthodox chemotherapy.

As of our last contact with this patient, the symptoms of his cancer had been absent for one and one-half years. The only treatment he has received is metabolic therapy including Laetrile.

APPENDIX

VM/SAC **PET** practice

remission of CANINE THYROID CARCINOMA following nitriloside therapy

George Browne, Jr., D.V.M.
Eureka Veterinary Hospital
4433 Highway 101 South
Eureka, California 95501

THE RATIONALE for using nitrilosides in cancer therapy was exhaustively reviewed in 1950.[1] Clinical reports of the beneficial effects of nitriloside in treatment of human cancer patients began to appear shortly thereafter. Reports from many parts of the world have described some degree of remission in terminal cancer patients following nitriloside therapy.[2-5] Toxic side effects commonly observed with other chemotherapeutic agents were reported to be minimal or not observed at all.

In this paper I report the use of amygdalin, the nitriloside most readily available in the United States, in treatment of thyroid carcinoma in a dog.

Case History

The subject of this report is a 5½-year-old male Pekingese dog. During routine physical examination accompanying an annual booster immunization, two firm nodular masses were palpated in the ventral cervical area. The masses were 1 cm. in diameter. No pain or inflammation were apparent.

Three weeks later, when this dog was examined again, the ventral cervical growths had enlarged to approximately 3 cm. in diameter. A narrow band of tissue connecting the two masses was palpable, with one lobe lying on either side of the trachea. A biopsy established the diagnosis of thyroid carcinoma. The dog showed no signs of illness.

When the dog was reexamined two weeks later, the growth had increased until it was interfering with deglutition. There were signs of anxiety and irritability alternating with periods of anorexia and depression.

A soft diet was prescribed and 500 mg. of amygdalin were administered intravenously on alternate days for a total of six injections. After this series of injections the growth had diminished in size, and a normal diet was reestablished. No difficulty in deglutition was encountered. The patient's attitude, activity and appetite had returned to normal. Treatments were reduced to twice-weekly intravenous injections of 500 mg. of amygdalin.

The twice-weekly regime was continued for one month, during which time the growth regressed to a size comparable to that palpated during the initial examination. Intravenous injections were discontinued and a daily maintenance dosage of 100 mg. of amygdalin per orum was established. This dosage has been continued for seven months.

A biopsy taken six and one-half months after the initiation of amygdalin therapy revealed no evidence of malignancy.

REFERENCES

1. Krebs, E.T., Jr.; *et al.*: The Unitarian or Trophoblastic Thesis of Cancer, *Med Rec. 163*:158-173; July 1950.
2. Navarro, M.D.: Laetrile—The Ideal Anti-Cancer Drug? *Santo Tomas J. Med. 9*:468-471; 1954.
3. Morrone, J.A.: Chemotherapy of Inoperable Cancer. *Exper. Med. & Surg. 4*, 1962.
4. Guidetti, E.: Observations Preliminaries Sur Quelques Cas de Cancer Traites Par Un Glycuronoside Cyanogenetique. *Acta Unio Internationales Contra Cancrum XI 2*: 156-158; 1955.
5. Nieper, H.A.: Critical Survey of the State of Cancer Research with Special Reference to Long Term Medical Therapy with Nitrilosides. Part I. *Krebsgeschehen 4,* 1972.

VM/SAC **PET** practice

remission of CANINE SQUAMOUS CELL CARCINOMA after nitriloside therapy

George Browne, Jr., DVM
Eureka Veterinary Hospital
4433 Highway 101 South
Eureka, California 95501

James D. Mortimer, DVM
4230 Canyon Lake Drive
Rapid City, South Dakota 57701

THE USE of nitrilosides in cancer therapy[1,2] has been the subject of heated controversy and extensive investigation. No nitriloside product has yet been cleared by the FDA for clinical use. In this paper we report apparently successful use of the nitriloside, amygdalin, to treat a squamous cell carcinoma in a dog.

The patient, a female mixed-breed dog weighing 15 lb (6. 75 kg), was approximately 10½ years old when first examined on December 12, 1972. At that time there was a tumor measuring 9 x 8 x 5 mm on the anterior aspect of the gum above the right upper canine tooth. The tumor was removed surgically and examined by a pathologist who classified it as a squamous cell carcinoma.

Seven days after surgery, cautery was required to control hemorrhaging.

The possibility of incomplete removal or metastasis of the tumor was considered. Therefore, on January 5, 1973, the dog was referred to the Veterinary Clinic, University of California at Davis, for evaluation and possible radiation therapy. The University Clinic reported as follows:

> *Our radiologic examination showed the squamous cell carcinoma of the right upper maxilla and dental arcade to be so invasive and to involve so much of the bone as to preclude treatment either with surgery or radiotherapy. The owners were so advised, and elected to keep the dog until such time as the tumor is making it so uncomfortable for the dog that they will have her euthanatized.*

On January 16, the owners consented to experimental treatment with amygdalin. The dog was given 1,600 mg of amygdalin intravenously on alternate days until 12 treatments had been given. When the last two injections were given, a small amount of amygdalin solution was infiltrated directly into the visible portions of the lesion.

On February 10, when intravenous treatments were discontinued, oral administration of amygdalin was started at a dose of 100 mg daily. After seven days without development of overt side effects the dose was increased to 400 mg daily.

On March 31, erosion of the gum and hard palate was noted. The lesion measured 1 cm.

On April 30, the appearance of the lesion had not changed.

On June 18, the eroded area was larger, involving more of the hard palate and measured 2 cm. Attempts to increase the oral dose of amygdalin to 500 to 700 mg per day resulted in vomiting immediately after administration of the drug. Dosage of 400 mg was renewed. During this period the mucous membranes appeared pale and the owner reported intermittent hemorrhaging from the lesion. The hematocrit was 21%. An oral hematinic (Vi-Sorbin®—Norden) was prescribed and given *per os* at the rate of 2 teaspoonsful daily.

On October 13th the lesion showed no further advance. The margins were necrotic and the center appeared to be filling with healthy granulation tissue.

By November 24, the lesion appeared to be completely healed. Administration of amygdalin was continued at 400 mg per day until January 16, 1974. The dosage was then reduced to 100 mg per day and kept at that level until June 3, 1975.

When examined on June 24, 1975, the dog was in good physical condition, active, and eating well. Some gingivitis and dental tartar were noted, and senile cataracts in the beginning stage were seen. Results of urinalysis, the CBC, and SGPT values were within normal limits. Blood urea nitrogen, lipase, and plasma protein values were slightly high.

The patient has been followed, and to date (April 1976) there has been no recurrence of the lesion.

REFERENCES

1. Navarro, M.D.: Laetrile—The Ideal Cancer Drug? *Santo Tomas J. Med.* 9:468-471; 1954.
2. Morrone, J.A.: Chemotherapy of Inoperable Cancer. *Exper. Med. & Surg.* 4:20, 299; 1962.

THE RICHARDSON CLINIC

514 KAINS AVENUE, ALBANY, CALIFORNIA 94706—TELEPHONE (415) 527-3020

A CORRECTIVE DIET FOR PATIENTS WITH A NEOPLASTIC DISEASE

Upon understanding what has happened that might have been responsible for a metabolic disease such as cancer, the tendency is to suddenly convert a lifetime of eating errors into a strict raw fruit and vegetable regimen. The family, wanting to do everything in their power to help a stricken loved one, may incorporate all of the weird and wonderful natural diets ever conceived by expert, friend, neighbor and loving relative. The only problem then appears to be that a digestive tract stubbornly accustomed to meat and potatoes screams in anguish when exposed to rabbit food. There is a weight loss and the patient who sees himself as a carrot stick topped with a sprig of parsley begins to wonder whether he's pleased that he heard about metabolic therapy.

So with this cautious introduction, let's make this new diet as simple as we can. Afer all, we know that certain vegetables and fruits will supplement nitrilosides, but we don't have to force feed them all at once because the metabolic regimen of vitamin injections will supply these in megavitamin doses.

Ours is a diet principally of fresh fruits, vegetables and grains. The one thing to be omitted from the diet is animal protein, including all meat (beef, pork, fish, poultry etc.) and all dairy products (milk, cream, cheese, etc.). Our previous diet permitted limited amounts of fish and poultry. However, experience has shown that many seriously ill patients are unable to handle this added metabolic load, especially where neoplastic involvement is extensive. We have also observed that the patients who have done consistently well are those who have followed the diet scrupulously and who have limited themselves to a minimal intake of animal protein.

There are two principal reasons for the exclusion of animal protein from the diet:

1) Of all major nutrients, proteins require the greatest amount of time and chemical energy for digestion and

assimilation. In a patient with advanced metabolic disease, it is preferable to supply the necessary amino acids in tablet form and to rely upon other sources (carbohydrates) for energy production.

2) If the digestive system (including the liver and pancreas) is not functioning properly—as is so often the case in cancer patients—animal proteins may be incompletely digested and undergo putrefaction. This means that some very toxic metabolic by-products, rather than the necessary amino acids, will be formed. These substances will further strain an already overloaded liver and interfere with vital biochemical processes in normal tissues.

Despite the omission of animal protein from the diet, you will receive an adequate intake of essential amino acids from the fruits and vegetables you eat and from the tablets (Ag/Pro) prescribed.

There are many commercial milk and meat substitutes available. Soy and coconut milk are to be especially recommended. A small amount of butter may be consumed; this is preferable to oleo. Hold salt intake to a minimum. Avoid chocolate and foods containing preservatives or artificial colorings. For the patient with advanced disease including liver involvement, the liver must be supported vigorously. Toxins should be eliminated from the diet. These include tobacco, alcohol, tranquilizers, sedatives, analgesics and coffee. Herbal teas are acceptable, however. Sufficient rest is important, and excessive exercise should be avoided.

With the exception of the above mentioned exclusions, most foods may be safely eaten. Include a variety of fresh fruits, vegetables, salads, nuts, natural juices, grains and oatmeals. Natural oils (safflower, peanut, olive, or sesame) may be used. Molasses, honey and maple sugar are preferable to refined sugar. Natural grain breads are obviously superior to white breads. Yeast is highly recommended. Assimilable fats and proteins are found in natural peanut butter. The diet emphasizes foods in "natural" form simply to preserve the true nutritive values of the vitamins and minerals present. Avoid extensive cooking (especially boiling) of vegetables.

Metabolic therapy is fairly standardized. But we do attempt to tailor it to each individual. On the average, a patient will receive twenty daily injections of multiple high dose vitamins with approximately six to nine grams of Laetrile or Vitamin B-17. Then there will be a tapering-off with three grams of Amygdalin and a reduced amount of the other vitamins by the intravenous or intramuscular route: three times weekly for one month; two times weekly for the next month; then at least once weekly wih oral supplementation until further notice, which is usually for eighteen months or so.

In addition, the patient is supplied with chelated minerals which we feel catalyse vitamin action. These chelates may be changed according to the results of the hair analysis. The word "chelation" means "claw"—more precisely, it is a way in which a mineral is tightly bound chemically to an amino acid or other organic molecule. It is felt that such bound minerals are better able to enter cells than non-chelated (free) minerals.

The following list is a summary of the standard oral supplements to the injection therapy. Please remember that these supplements will be adjusted somewhat for individual cases according to needs and tolerance.

1) Pancreatic Enzyme Tablets—two to four tablets, four times daily. Increased flatulence (gas) may occur with an increased or lowered dosage. This dosage may be adjusted according to how a patient responds.

2) Vitamin B-15 (Pangamic Acid)—50mg. three times daily. Pangamic Acid aids the liver in the detoxification processes as a transmethylating agent. It also increases the oxygen uptake potential of the tissues.

3) Vitamin C—750mg. to 2,000mg. daily.

4) Amino Acid Tablets (Ag/Pro)—three to nine tablets daily to compensate for reduced intake of animal protein.

5) Chelated Minerals—dosage dependent upon extent of deficiency revealed by hair analysis. The following minerals are available in chelated form: Calcium, Magnesium, Iron, Manganese, and Zinc.

6) Therapeutic Vitamins and Minerals (Supergran)—one or two capsules daily. This supplies the necessary Vitamin A, B-Complex, additional Vitamin C, and Vitamin D in sufficient doses. Included also are several essential trace minerals.

7) Vitamin E—800 I.U. to 1,200 I.U. daily.

8) Additional Vitamins and Minerals—to be recommended where necessary in special cases. These may include any of a wide variety of vitamins, minerals, chelates, amino acids, or other food factors.

Occasionally, the digestive tract of a severely ill patient will rebel at the ingestion of vitamins and minerals in a form to which it is not accustomed. If this be so, simply back off and start slowly, adding each one separately and gradually increasing the dose until one achieves maximum intake compatible with a feeling of well being.

While the diet may seem unduly restrictive, you should remember that degenerative diseases—especially cancer—must be fought as aggressively and quickly as possible by non-toxic methods before a disease progresses to an irreversible stage. No one can force you to adhere rigidly to any diet. This must be a matter of personal discipline and commitment. However, the ultimate outcome of the entire treatment regimen will depend in large part upon your full cooperation and understanding of these issues.

JOHN A. RICHARDSON, M.D.
514 KAINS AVENUE
ALBANY, CALIFORNIA 94706
TELEPHONE 527-3020

Dear Patient:

I am writing this letter to avoid any misunderstanding concerning your bioassay test results. The bioassay result reported together with this letter is a measure of nitrogen balance and is not a diagnostic test for cancer or malignant disease. However, together with other laboratory test data, it does provide us with additional information concerning your state of health. The bioassay gives us some idea of the rate of cell division in the body (including, of course, normal as well as abnormal cells), as determined by one measurement of nitrogen metabolism

To simplify matters we use the following scale as a general guide to interpretation of results:

17.0 or less	=	within normal limits
17.1 - 24.0	=	borderline
24.1 or more	=	outside normal limits

Nevertheless, I must emphasize that results must be interpreted together with information obtained from other blood and urine studies, X-rays, medical history, physical examination and previous medical treatment. The same is true for any test result - it can not be considered alone. It is possible for a normal (presumably healthy) individual to show an elevated bioassay result; conversely, a patient with malignant disease may show a bioassay within normal limits (perhaps as a result of recent chemotherapy and/or radiation). If either situation is the case, we recommend repeating the test at a later date.

I hope that this brief explanation has served to clarify the results being reported to you at this time. Please consult with this office if you have any further questions concerning this test or any other tests performed in your case.

Sincerely,

John A. Richardson, M.D.

John A. Richardson, M.D.

Above is a reproduction of a letter sent to Richardson Clinic patients along with results of their urine bioassay test. Prior to November, 1976, a different laboratory was used and, therefore, the lab results in this book which were done before that date should be read using the following lab normals: 0-15, negative; 15-20, borderline; 20 + , positive.

LABORATORY TESTS

Table Abbreviations

gm. = gram
μg. = microgram
μμg. = micromicrogram
ng. = nanogram
pg. = picogram

mm. = millimeter
cu.mm. = cubic millimeter
mU. = milliunit
μU. = microunit
mEq. = milliequivalent

μ = micron or micrometer
cuμ = cubic microns
I.U. = international unit
L. = liter

NORMAL VALUES—HEMATOLOGY (BLOOD STUDIES)

Determination	Normal Value	Clinical Significance (Partial List)
Erythrocyte count (Red blood cells, RBC)	Male: 4,600,000-6,200,000 per cu. mm. Female: 4,200,000-5,400,000 per cu. mm.	Increased in severe diarrhea and dehydration. Decreased in all anemias, leukemia, and after hemorrhage, when blood volume has been restored
Hematocrit	Male: 42-50% Female: 40-48%	Decreased in severe anemias, or acute massive blood loss. Increased in erythrocytosis of any cause, and in dehydration or hemoconcentration asssociated with shock.

Hemoglobin	Male: 13-16 gm./100 ml. Female: 12-14 gm./100 ml.	Decreased in various anemias, severe or prolonged hemorrhage, and with excessive fluid intake. Increased in chronic obstructive pulmonary diseases, failure of oxygenation because of congestive heart failure, and normally, in people living at high altitudes.
Leukocyte alkaline phosphatase	Score of 40-100	Decreased in chronic myelocytic leukemia and chronic lymphocytic leukemia. Increased in nonleukemic leukocytosis and myeloproliferative diseases.
Leukocyte count (white blood cells, WBC)	Total: 5,000-10,000 cu. mm.	Elevated in acute infectious diseases. Elevated in acute leukemia, following menstruation, and following surgery or trauma. Depressed in aplastic anemia, and by toxic agents, such as chemotheraptutic agents used in treating malignancy.
Platelet count	200,000-350,000 per cu. mm.	Increased with chronic granulocytic leukemia, hemoconcentration. Decreased in acute leukemia, aplastic anemia, and during cancer chemotherapy.

NORMAL BLOOD OR SERUM VALUES

Determination	Normal Adult Values	Clinical Significance (Partial List) (Increased)	(Decreased)
Bilirubin	Total: 0.1-1.0 mg./100 ml. Direct: 0.1-0.2 mg./100 ml. Indirect: 0.1-0.8 mg./100 ml.	Hemolytic anemia (indirect) Biliary obstruction Hepatocellular damage	
Bromsulfophthalein (BSP)	Less than 5% retention in 45 min.	Acute hepatic diseases	
Gamma glutamyl transpeptidase	Men: less than 45 I.U./L. Women: less than 30 I.U./L.	Hepatobiliary disease Drug therapy damage	
Glucose	65-110 mg./100 ml.	Diabetes Hyperthyroidism Cerebral lesions Infections	Extensive hepatic damage

Isocitric dehydrogenase	50-180 units	Hepatitis, cirrhosis Obstructive jaundice Metastatic carcinoma to the liver	
Lactic dehydrogenase (LDH)	90-200 mU./ml.	Untreated pernicious anemia Pulmonary infarction Liver disease	
Phosphatase, acid	0-2 units/ml. (Shinowara-Jones-Reinhart units)	Carcinoma of prostate	
Phosphatase, alkaline	4-17 King-Amstrong units/ml.	Conditions reflecting increased osteoblastic activity of bone Liver disease	
Protein, total	6-8 gm./100 ml.	Hemoconcentration Shock	Malnutrition Hemorrhage
Albumin	3.5-5 gm./100 ml.	Multiple myeloma (globulin fraction)	Proteinuria
Globulin	1.5-3 gm./100 ml.	Chronic infections (globulin)	

NORMAL BLOOD OR SERUM VALUES (Continued)

Determination	Normal Adult Values	Clinical Significance (Partial List) (Increased)	(Decreased)
Testosterone	Adult males: 400-1200 ng./100 ml. Adult females: 30-150 ng./100 ml.	Females: Polycystic ovary Virilizing tumors	Males: Orchidectomy for neoplastic disease of the prostate or breast Estrogen therapy Hepatic cirrhosis
Transaminase (SGOT)	15-45 units/ml.	Skeletal muscle disease Liver disease	
Transaminase (SGPT)	5-36 units/ml.	Same conditions as SGOT, but increase is more marked in liver disease than SGOT	
Urea nitrogen	10-20 mg./100 ml.	Obstructive uropathy	Severe hepatic failure
Uric acid	1-6 mg./100 ml.	Gouty arthritis Acute leukemia Lymphomas treated by chemotherapy	

NORMAL VALUES—URINE CHEMISTRY

Determination	Normal Adult Values	Clinical Significance (Partial List) (Increased)	(Decreased)
Alpha amino nitrogen	64-199 mg./24 hrs.	Leukemia Other metabolic diseases	
Ammonia	20-70 mEq./L. 0.6 gm./L.	Cirrhosis and other destructive diseases of the liver	
Bile melanin	Zero	Advanced melanoma	
Chorionic gonadotropin	Zero	Pregnancy Chorionepithelioma	
Creatine	Less than 100 mg./24 hrs.	Fever Carcinoma of liver	
Creatinine	1-2 gm./24 hrs.		Advanced degeneration of kidneys Leukemia

NORMAL VALUES—URINE CHEMISTRY (Continued)

Determination	Normal Adult Values	Clinical Significance (Partial List) (Increased)	(Decreased)
Bile melanin	Zero	Advanced melanoma	
Estrogens, total	Female: Onset of menstruation: 4-25 μg./24 hr. Ovulation peak: 28-99 μg./24 hr. Luteal peak: 22-105 μg./24 hr. Menopausal women: 1.4-19.6 μg./24 hr. Male: 5-18 μg./24 hrs.	Hyperestrogenism due to gonadal or adrenal neoplasm	Primary or secondary amenorrhea

THE

DISPENSATORY

OF THE

UNITED STATES OF AMERICA.

BY GEORGE B. WOOD, M.D.,

PROFESSOR OF MATERIA MEDICA AND PHARMACY IN THE PHILADELPHIA COLLEGE OF PHARMACY, MEMBER OF THE AMERICAN PHILOSOPHICAL SOCIETY, &c., &c.;

AND

FRANKLIN BACHE, M.D.,

PROFESSOR OF CHEMISTRY IN THE PHILADELPHIA COLLEGE OF PHARMACY, ONE OF THE SECRETARIES OF THE AMERICAN PHILOSOPHICAL SOCIETY, &c., &c.

PHILADELPHIA:

PUBLISHED BY GRIGG & ELLIOT,

NO. 9 NORTH FOURTH STREET.

1833.

Title page from an 1833 reference volume in which amygdalin is described as a common treatment for a wide range of diseases and disorders. Clearly, it is not a "New Drug" as the FDA claims.

Glossary

ab·dom·i·no·per·ne'al re·sec'tion. The large bowel is cut above the cancer and the open end brought out of the abdomen. The tumor and all the bowel from the tumor to the anus is removed and the anus sewn shut. The patient then has bowel movements from an opening on his abdomen.

ac·e·tab'u·lum. The rounded cavity on the external surface of the innominate bone which receives head of femur. The part of the hip bone which comes in contact with the upper leg bone.

ad·e·no·ac·an·tho'ma. Adenocarcinoma in which some cells have undergone squamous metaplasia. A cancer cell that looks scale-like under a microscope.

ad·e·no·car·cin·o'ma. A malignant adenoma arising from epithelium of a glandular organ. A cancer which has its origin in the covering of an internal or external surface of the body.

ad·e·no' ma·tous. Pert. to adenomas. Pertaining to tumors arising from coverings of an internal or external surface of the body.

ad·e·nop'a·thy. Swelling and morbid change in lymph nodes; glandular disease. Swollen glands.

a'la. An expanded or winglike structure or appendage. The ala of the nose is the cartilage, the bone-like material which gives the nose its shape.

al'ky·lat·ing a'gent. 1. A substance which introduces an alkyl radical into a compound in place of a hydrogen atom. 2. A chemotherapeutic agent capable of destroying human cells (cancer and non-cancer cells) at all stages in the cell's life cycle.

a·mel·a·not'ic. Without melanin; unpigmented.

an·a·plas′tic. Pert. to anaplasia. The change of a cell to a more-primitive type, often associated with cancer.
ap′i·cal. Pert. to the apex.
as·tro·cy·to′ma. Tumor formed from astrocytes. Astrocytes are star-shaped connective tissue cells in the brain and spinal cord.
a·typ′ism. Non-typical. Deviation from normal.
ax′il·lar·y. Pert. to the axilla. The armpit area.
bil·i·ru′bin. The orange-colored or yellowish pigment in bile.
car·ci·no′ma. An epithelial cell new growth or malignant tumor, enclosed in connective tissue, and tending to infiltrate and give rise to metastases. Cancer.
ceph′a·lad. Toward the head; e.g., the elbow is 9-11 inches cephalad (closer to the head) to the wrist.
cer′vi·cal. 1. Of, pert. to, or in the region of the neck. 2. Pert. to the cervix of an organ, as the cervix uteri.
cer′vi·cal ver′te·brae. First seven bones of the spinal column.
co·li′tis. Inflammation of the colon.
co·los′to·my. Incision of the colon for purpose of making a more or less permanent fistula between the bowel and the abdominal wall. A surgical procedure after which the patient has bowel movements from a hole in the abdomen.
col·pos′co·py. Examination of the fornices of the vagina and cervix uteri. An examination of the female organs, by instrument.
com′mis·sure. The coming together of two structures, as the lips, eyelids, or vocal cords.
co·ni·za′tion. Excision of a cone of tissue, as of the mucous membrane of the cervix. The purpose of removing the cone of tissue is to see if the tissue is cancerous.
cu·ret′tings. Material surgically scraped from a body cavity, such as the bladder or uterus.
cys·ti′tis. Inflammation of the bladder usually occurring secondarily to infections of associated organs (kidney, prostate, urethral). May be acute or chronic.
cys·to·scop′ic exam. Examination of the inside of the bladder by means of a lighted instrument.
cys·to·u·re·thro′scop·y. Examination of the posterior urethra and urinary bladder.
de·hy·dro′gen·ase. An enzyme which catalyzes the oxidation of a specific substance, causing it to give up its hydrogen.

dys·pla′sia. Abnormality of development.

dis′tal sig′moid. End of the large bowel near the rectum.

di·ver·tic·u·lo′sis. Diverticula in the colon without inflammation or symptoms. An outpouching of the intestinal wall. These are usually seen as many tiny finger-like or balloon-like bumps on what should be a smooth gut wall.

dor′sal. 1. Pert. to the back. 2. Indicating a position toward a rear part.

duc′tal. Pertaining to a narrow tubular vessel or channel, esp. one serving to convey secretions from a gland, e.g. the milk ducts of a female breast.

ech′o·gram. A picture produced by sound waves. Echography is the use of ultrasonic technique to obtain a photograph of the echo produced when sound waves are reflected from tissues of different density.

em·bry·on′al. Pert. to or resembling an embryo.

en·do·cer′vi·cal. Pert. to the endocervix, the lining of the canal of the cervix.

en·do·me′tri·um. The mucous membrane lining the inner surface of the uterus

ep·i·the′li·al. Pert. to or composed of epithelium, the covering of internal and external surfaces of the body.

e·soph·a·gi′tis. Inflammation of the esophagus.

e·ti·ol′o·gy. The study of the causes of disease.

ex·ci′sion. An act of cutting away or taking out.

fun′gat·ing. Growing rapidly like a fungus, applied to certain tumors

gran·u·lo′ma·ta. Granular tumors usually of lymph cells (as in Hodgkin's Disease) or epithelial cells.

gy·ne·col′o·gist. Physician who specializes in diseases of the female reproductive system.

hem·a·tu′ri·a. Blood in the urine.

he·mo·lyt′ic. Pert. to the breaking down of red blood cells.

hemo·sta′sis. 1. Arrest of bleeding or of circulation. 2. Stagnation of blood.

hem·a·tol′o·gy. The science concerned with blood and the blood-forming tissues.

he·mat′o·crit. 1. Centrifuge for separating solids from plasma in the blood. 2. The volume of erythrocytes packed by centrifugation in a given volume of blood.

her·ni·orrh′a·phy. Surgical operation for repair of hernia. Hernia is the pushing of an organ or part of an organ past the wall of the body cavity which normally contains it.

hi·lar. Depression in an organ where the blood vessels enter, as in the kidney, lungs, and various glands.

his·to·cy·to'ma. A tumor containing histocytes. Histocytes are tissue cells.

hy·per·pig·men·ta'tion. Abnormal (too much) coloring, usually of the skin.

hy·per'tro·phy. Increased size of an organ, or of the body, due to abnormal growth.

hy·po·gly·ce'mi·a. Deficiency of sugar in the blood. A condition in which the glucose in the blood is abnormally low.

il'e·al. Pert. to the ileum, part of the small bowel.

il'i·ac crest. The high point of the hip bone which can be felt just below the waist.

in'gui·nal. Pert. to the region of the groin.

in·va'sive. Entering nearby tissue.

jug·u·lo·di·gas'tric. The neck area.

la'bi·al. Pert. to the folds of tissue on either side of the vaginal opening.

lap·ar·ot'o·my. The surgical opening of the abdomen; an abdominal operation.

lar·yn'ge·al. Pert. to the larynx, the vocal cords.

lob'u·lat·ed. Consisting of lobes or lobules. 2. Pert. to lobes or lobules. 3. Resembling lobes.

loc'u·lat·ed. Containing or divided into loculi, i.e., small cavities.

lym·phad·e·nop'a·thy. Disease of the lymph nodes.

lym·phan'gi·o·grams. A procedure that allows the doctor to look for disease (usually cancer) in the lymph system without having to perform surgery. A dye, which shows up in X-rays, is injected into the lymphatic vessels at the hands or feet, and a series of X-rays is taken following the path the dye travels.

lym·phat'ic. Of or pert. to lymph vessels and nodes.

lym·pho·cy'tic. Pertaining to lymphocytes — lymph cells or white blood cells.

lym·pho'ma. A general term for growth of cancer tissue in the lymphatic system. This group (of cancers) includes Hodgkin's Disease, lymphosarcoma, and malignant lymphoma.

lym·pho·sar·co'ma. A malignant disease of lymphatic tissue. Clinically may be quite similar to Hodgkin's disease.

mam'mo·gram. An X-ray picture of the breast.

mas·tec'to·my (radical). Removal of a breast and the

muscles underneath the breast down to the chest wall; also includes removal of the lymph nodes under the arm.

me'di·al. 1. Pert. to middle. 2. Nearer the medial plane.

me·di·as·ti'nal. Rel. to the mediastinum.

me·di·as·ti'num. 1. A septum or cavity between two principal portions of an organ. 2. The folds of the pleura and intervening space between right and left lung. 3. The area between the right and left lung.

mel·a·no'ma. A malignant, pigmented mole or tumor. The most serious skin cancer.

mes'en·ter·y. 1. A peritoneal fold, encircling the greater part of the small intestines and connecting the intestine to the post-abdominal wall. 2. A thin fold of flesh that holds the gut in place at the back of the abdomen.

mes·o·ne·phro'ma. A relatively rare tumor derived from mesonephric cells developing in reproductive organs, esp. ovary or genital tract. Mesonephric cells refer to cells in the embryo (the unborn child) which will later become part of the reproductive system.

mes·o·the·li·o'ma. Tumor (cancer) starting in the lining of a body cavity.

met·a·bol'ic. Pert. to metabolism. Metabolism is the sum of all physical and chemical changes that take place within the body; all energy and material changes that occur within the cells. It includes both the use, and the breakdown and elimination, of materials by the body.

me·tas'ta·sis. 1. The appearance of a second cancer in a different location from the first. 2. Change in location of a disease or of its manifestations or transfer from one organ or part to another not directly connected. (The chance of survival after metastasis is practically zero.)

met·a·stat'ic. Pert. to metastasis.

mu'cin. A glyco-protein found in mucus.

mu'co·cele. 1. Enlargement of the lacrimal sac. 2. A mucous cyst (A cyst is a closed sac or pouch which is walled and contains fluid, semifluid, or solid material. It is usually an abnormal structure.)

mu·co'sa. Mucous membrane.

mus·cu·la'ris. Muscular layer of an organ or tubule.

my·e·log'en·ous. Producing or originating in bone marrow.

ne·cro'sis. Death of areas of tissue or bone surrounded by healthy parts.

ne·crot'ic. Rel. to death of a portion of tissue.

ne'o·plasm. A new and abnormal formation of tissue, as a tumor or growth. It serves no useful function but grows at the expense of the healthy organism. Frequently used as a substitute for the word cancer. It is more accurate to say malignant neoplasm when referring to cancer.

ne'o·plas·tic. Pert. to, or of the nature of, new, abnormal tissue formation; usually refers to cancer.

node. 1. A knot, knob, protuberance, or swelling. 2. A small rounded organ or structure, as a lymph node.

oc·cip'i·tal. Concerning the back part of the head.

or'i·fice. Mouth, entrance, or outlet to any aperture.

os·te·o·blas'tic. Refers to the osteoblast, a cell which is involved in forming bones.

pal'li·a·tive. 1. Serving to relieve or alleviate, without curing. 2. An agent which alleviates or eases.

pal'pa·ble. Perceptible, esp. by touch. Usually refers to a lump, or a body organ which can be felt only when involved in disease. (A doctor would not palpate the nose; he would feel it. He would, however, palpate the armpit to see if there were swollen glands present.)

pap'il·lar·y. 1. Concerning a nipple or papilla. 2. Resembling or composed of papillae.

para·cla·vic·u·lar. Around or near the collar bone (the clavicle.).

para·me'tri·al. Around or near the uterus.

par·a·tra'che·al. Around or near the windpipe (the trachea).

pa·ri'e·tes. Walls of an organ or hollow part.

per·i·hi'lar. 1. Around or near the bronchi, the large tubes through which air enters and leaves lungs 2. Also, around or near the notch (the *hilum*) of the kidney.

per·i·ne'al. Concerning, or situated on, the perineum. The perineum is the area on the outside of the body between the vulva and the anus in a female or between the scrotum and anus in a male.

per·i·to·ne'um. 1. The serous membrane reflected over the viscera and lining the abdominal cavity. 2. Thin tissue lining the abdomen.

phos'pha·tase. One of the group of enzymes which catalyzes the hydrolysis of phosphoric acid esters. They are of importance in absorption and metabolism of carbohydrates, nucleotides, and phospholipids and are essential in the calcification of bone.

proc′tos·cope. Instrument for inspection of the inside of the rectum.

rad′i·cal. 1. A group of atoms acting as a single unit, passing without change from one compound to another, but not able to exist in a free state. 2. Anything that reaches the root or origin; original. 3. Radical surgery is that surgery in which large amounts of tissue or bone are removed.

rads. Rad is an abbreviation for radiation absorbed dose. It is the unit of measure used in calculating how much radiation a body part will receive.

re′nal. 1. Pert. to the kidney. 2. Shaped like a kidney.

re·sect′. Cut off or cut out a portion of a structure or organ, as to cut off the end of a bone or remove a segment of the intestine.

re·tic′u·lo·cyte. A red blood cell containing a network of granules or filaments representing an immature stage in development.

re·tic′u·lum. A network.

rhab·do·myo·sar·co′ma. Cancer arising from muscle tissue which appears rod-shaped under a microscope.

sar·co′ma. Cancer arising from underlying tissue: muscle, bone, and other connective tissue. May affect the bones, bladder, kidneys, liver, lungs, parotids, and spleen.

scir′rhous. Hard, like a scirrhus. A hard cancerous tumor caused by overgowth of fibrous tissue.

SGOT. Abbr. for serum glutamic-oxalacetic transaminase. (See appendix.)

sig′moid. The last part of the large bowel just before the rectum.

sig·moid·o′scopy. An instrument for examining the inside of the large bowel as far as the signoid.

si′tus. (in si-tu). In situ means in position or in place. Cancer *in situ* refers to a small cancer which has not yet eaten into nearby tissue.

squa′mous. Scale-like.

ste·no′sis. Constriction or narrowing of a passage or orifice. Stenosis can be caused by the hard fibrous scar tissue which can be formed following radiation.

sub·cu·ta′ne·ous. Beneath or to be introduced beneath the skin.

te·nes′mus. Spasm of the anal or urinary outlet with pain and the almost constant feeling of the need to empty the bowel or bladder.

tho·ra′cic. Pert. to the chest or thorax.

trans·am′i·nase. An enzyme that catalyzes transamination. (See the appendix, under laboratory studies.)

trans·u·re′thral. Pert. to an operation performed through the urethra.

tu·me·fac′tion. 1. A swelling. 2. Act of swelling or the state of being swollen. 3. A tumor. (The word tumefaction is used frequently in place of the word cancer or malignant tumefaction.)

u′re·ter. One of two tubes carrying urine from the kidneys to the bladder.

u·re′thra. The tube that carries urine from the bladder to the outside of the body.

u′ter·ine. Pert. to the uterus.

val·lec′u·la. A depression or crevice.

ver′te·bra. Any one of the 33 bony segments of the spinal column. The 33 vertebrae (starting from the neck) are comprised of 7 cervical, 12 thoracic (or dorsal), 5 lumbar, 5 sacral, and 4 coccygeal.

ves′i·cal. Pert. to or shaped like a bladder.

vil′lous. Pert. to or furnished with villi or with fine hairlike extensions.

W.B.C. Abbr. for white blood count; white blood cells.

ze′ro·gram. A type of X-ray. This special X-ray shows all tissue in bas relief.

ze·ro·mam′mo·gram. A type of X-ray of the breast.

Index

ABOUT THE AUTHORS

DR. JOHN RICHARDSON has been in the forefront of the Laetrile controversy since 1972. He has challenged the FDA in and out of court in his continuing battle to secure the right of physician and patient to reject orthodox cancer treatments—in which they have little confidence—and use nutritional therapy instead.

Dr. Richardson received his Doctor of Medicine degree from the University of Rochester School of Medicine in New York. He completed his internship plus a one-year fellowship in medicine at the Mary Imogene Bassett Hospital in Cooperstown, New York. In 1952 he was awarded the title of *Diplomate* by the National Board of Medical Examiners. In that same year he received his license to practice medicine and surgery in the state of New York. In August of 1954 he was certified by the state of California and he has conducted his practice in the San Francisco Bay area since that time.

PAT GRIFFIN is a native Californian, who grew up in Michigan. She was graduated from the University of Michigan, School of Nursing, in June, 1953. After working as a psychiatric nurse and in public health nursing, she returned to college in 1973 and received her Bachelor of Science degree in nursing from Mount Saint Mary's College in West Los Angeles in June, 1975. She lives in southern California with her husband, G. Edward Griffin, and their children.

ROBERT SAM ANSON was a correspondent for *Time* for six years. He reported from Chicago, New York, Los Angeles and Indochina. Mr. Anson is currently Executive Producer for Special Events for public television station WNET in New York and Senior Writer of *New*

Times magazine. His articles have also appeared in *Harper's*, the *Atlantic*, *Columbia Journalism Review* and *Ms*. He is the author of two books, *McGovern: A Biography* and *"They've Killed the President!" The Search for the Murderers of John F. Kennedy*.